CW01656517

Joanne's Story

Today I Chose to Smile

Margo Pentland

Published by Neetah Books

First printing: May 2020

Printed by Ingram.

All photographs are courtesy of Margo Pentland.

A CIP catalogue for this title is available from the British Library.

ISBN: 978-1-908898-43-2

This book is also available in Kindle

www.neetahbooks.com

DEDICATION

To Joanne
For all we went through together
and the love we shared xx

ACKNOWLEDGEMENTS

Thomas Starlz – the man who carried out the world's first liver transplant

Peter Raine – the man who carried out Joanne's Kasai operation in 1979 and gave us hope

Peter Johnson – the man who carried out Joanne's first and second liver transplants in Cambridge in 1990

Jim Powell and K K Madhavan – the men who carried out Joanne's third liver transplant in Edinburgh in 2007

The Liver Transplant team in Edinburgh – for taking care of Joanne over many years. Special thanks to Dr Ken Simpson and the transplant co-ordinators – you were amazing.

Grateful thanks to every single person who is involved in the care of donors and their families, recipients and their families before and after organ transplantation

Organ donors and their families everywhere

Rev. Ian Miller for support, help and encouragement throughout the process of writing this book

Paul Murdoch for agreeing to publish the book

Joe and Neil and Liz – for their unending support

Stuart, Leigh, Joseph and Kara

My friends and family who have continued to support me. It means so much.

Joanne's friends – the girls (and boys) who love and miss her and make sure I know.

1

John and I were married in early 1976. We settled into married life, and when I became pregnant with our first child in 1978, we were over the moon. Like many young couples though, our first pregnancy ended in heartbreak when I miscarried our baby in June of that year.

It wasn't long before I became pregnant again, and on 17th September 1979 Joanne was born at Vale of Leven Hospital Maternity Unit. This pregnancy was uneventful considering my recent history, up until around two weeks before my due date. At my GP's ante natal clinic on 13th September, my blood pressure was unusually high, so my doctor phoned the maternity hospital explaining that we had discussed this and agreed that, since it was late Friday afternoon, I should go home and spend the weekend in bed and attend the hospital first thing on Monday morning. The consultant, however, had other ideas. Although there would be no consultant on duty in the hospital over the weekend, he insisted that I was to be admitted to hospital that day and spend the weekend under the watchful eye of junior doctors and nursing staff. Reluctantly I went home, packed a bag, and was driven to the hospital by my husband John. Over the weekend I was not allowed to put a foot over the bed. Staff were there to assist with washing me and on hand with a bedpan when required. Within myself I felt absolutely fine, and not at all unwell. Monday morning, I was seen by the consultant during his ward round. When he examined me he discovered that I was haemorrhaging internally and immediately set the wheels in motion for me to have an emergency C section. And so Joanne was born two weeks early at 12.20 pm on Monday 17th September 1979.

After the birth we were given a private room and waited on hand and foot. The consultant told me we were both "very lucky ladies to be alive", and although he was well known locally by staff and patients alike for being a formidable character, he was amazingly kind and we honestly couldn't have been treated better. As he had just saved both our lives, I couldn't praise him highly enough.

Over the next few days, Joanne developed what looked like a lump near her eye. It turned out to be a blocked tear duct, so she had to stay in hospital for treatment which was given by 7 daily injections over a two week period. The injections were given alternately on each buttock, at regular intervals. Even then, she didn't make a fuss. An insight on how she would be throughout her life as a hospital patient. Joanne was transferred to the Baby Care Unit for this treatment after I was discharged. We visited every day, spending time feeding and changing her, but couldn't wait to get her home.

During one of our visits, one of the nursery nurses mentioned to me that she had noticed Joanne was looking a bit jaundiced and she had brought this to the attention of the doctors. They weren't unduly worried about it but if it didn't subside in the next few days they would give her a special type of light treatment called Phototherapy, designed to lower the bilirubin levels in her blood.

At that time, there was always a Paediatric Consultant from the Sick Children's Hospital in Glasgow who paid a visit to the baby care unit once a week. When Joanne was 4 weeks old, the Consultant spoke with John and I and said she was concerned that, although Joanne's eye problem had been successfully cleared, her jaundice was not going away despite the phototherapy treatment. The Consultant explained that the jaundice could be caused by one of three problems . Two were treatable, but the third was very rare and unlikely to be the cause so she didn't go into that option in any great detail other than to say that it was "unthinkable and untreatable".

At 5 weeks old Joanne was transferred to the Sick Children's Hospital for investigative scans, tests and surgery if necessary. I was allowed to stay with her in a private room and look after her for the first time – just like any new mum only in a hospital environment - but after a week I had to go home to allow them to carry out more extensive tests and prepare Joanne for investigative surgery.

On the day of her surgery, I kept myself busy at home while John went to work to keep his mind off things. He was the one designated to make the phone call to the hospital that day to see how Joanne was after the op., and just after lunch time he phoned me to say that he had phoned the hospital, but they wouldn't give him any information other than she was back from theatre and that we were to go up to speak to the surgeon. We tried to convince ourselves that this was all perfectly normal, but we both had a bad feeling. John insisted that he would just jump in the car and go up himself, without waiting for me to get myself ready. What seemed like a lifetime later, he arrived home. One look was enough for me to fear the worst. My mind was racing. I thought something had happened during or after the surgery and our daughter had died. John's eyes were red from crying. I guessed he had been crying all the way home and I don't think he knew how to begin to tell me what had happened.

To this day, I just remember words that I had never heard before - biliary atresia, situs inversus, aortic stenosis. These were the three main medical problems they had discovered during the exploratory procedure but there were others including no gall bladder, and no fully grown spleen, and some other defects which they said were minor in comparison to the main health issues she had.

Biliary Atresia happens when the liver's bile ducts – tubes that carry bile out of the liver - are either missing or blocked. The causes of biliary atresia remain unknown, but when bile can't leave the liver it causes liver damage and among children, it is the most common reason for liver failure. Life expectancy is 9 months if untreated.

Situs Inversus is a congenital condition where the major visceral organs are reversed or mirrored from their normal positions. Because Joanne's organs were reversed below her heart, her "wiring" was very complex. This condition often proves fatal.

Aortic Stenosis is one of the most common and most serious heart valve disease problems, and can often be a complication of Situs Inversus. Although aortic stenosis can be present without any symptoms for many years, it can weaken the heart and require surgery.

The surgeon, Professor Dan Young, told John that there was no cure for Joanne's liver condition, and that attempts at performing an operation called the Kasai, which may extend her life expectancy to around 2 years, had never been successful in Scotland, so they no longer carried out the operation. He also said that with her complications it was unlikely that she would have a life expectancy of 2 years even with the operation, and that as she was "wired up wrong " it would make the operation very difficult to perform on Joanne. So he ruled it out as an option.

We learned over the years that most hospital doctors and surgeons in Britain were not keen on performing pioneering surgery or treatments on young children at that time. But my view was – as a desperate mum of a very sick baby – someone has to be first to have a successful outcome. We asked if there was any treatment in any hospital anywhere in the world that could help our daughter, but were met with negative responses to all of our questions. We were distraught. Our baby was going to die, and there was nothing we could do about it. Professor Young was not willing to consider any form of treatment for Joanne, and said that once she had fully recovered from the surgery, we were to take her home and make her as comfortable as possible.

We left the hospital after going up to visit Joanne and made our way home. I didn't want to tell anyone about our discussion with the surgeon. I didn't want people feeling sorry for Joanne, or for her to be put in the spotlight. I wanted to take her home and try to make her life as normal as possible for however long she had. Maybe that's just a mother trying to protect her young, but John took a different view. He said that we should tell family at the very least as we would need their support. Of course, he was right. We went to my mum's to break the news to her and afterwards John went back to work to lock up the school where he worked as janitor. The head teacher, Mrs Good, was still there when he got back to the school that afternoon, and when she asked how things had gone, John found himself blurting out to her that things were not looking good for Joanne. He ended up in her office, with her listening carefully to him relating what we had been told. Mrs Good asked John if we would like her to get in touch with the School Chaplain, Reverend Bill MacFarlane. Before he left her office, John telephoned me at mum's and we agreed that we would both like to speak with Mr MacFarlane. Although I was 28 years old at the time, I hadn't been a regular attender at church since my days of going to Sunday School as a youngster growing up in Renton. But instinctively, I felt that this was the right thing to do. We needed divine intervention!

2

Not long after John arrived home from work, Mr MacFarlane telephoned me and asked if it would be ok to visit. I said of course, and shortly after he came to the house to speak with us. Strangely, I felt while Mr Macfarlane was listening and talking to us that everything would be ok. It was a weird feeling – almost surreal. Before he left, Mr MacFarlane asked if we would like him to baptise Joanne at the hospital. Having Joanne baptised at the earliest possible moment just felt right so we said yes.

The next day we made arrangements to meet Mr MacFarlane later to have Joanne christened that evening with the hospital doctor's approval to do so after visiting hours. Word seemed to have got round on the ward about Joanne's illness. Some mothers were offering words of comfort or sympathy, but others were saying things like "poor you, at least even although my child has cancer, I have hope". It wasn't the nicest thing to hear – words I have never forgotten.

That evening we returned to the hospital with Mr Macfarlane to have our baby christened. Joanne was lying naked in an incubator except for a nappy and was wired up to all sorts of monitors in the high dependency section of the baby ward. It was November time so it was dark outside, and inside the room was dimly lit. It was very quiet and peaceful except for the sound of the various machines that were keeping the small babies alive.

I had brought up a Christening shawl that had been passed down through the family, but Joanne never got to wear it. I was only allowed to hold Joanne's hand through the hole at the side of the incubator. Mr MacFarlane had a bottle with Holy Water in it, and he poured some of it into what looked like a sugar bowl! (After his passing many years later, his wife gave us the very bowl that he used that night. He had kept it for all those years in a small box, wrapped in tissue paper, with a small tag that read "Joanne's christening bowl"). Despite the circumstances, Joanne's Christening was just perfect. Mr

MacFarlane's words were so meaningful and straight from the heart. Each word spoken was specific to Joanne's circumstances, and was said with such conviction that I couldn't help but believe that God would make things right for her.

Mr MacFarlane – and his wife Margaret – became a very big part of our future lives. From not knowing us from Adam, he became a regular visitor to our home, visiting every second Wednesday for the next four years without fail! He sure had a soft spot for Joanne, and as for her, well she just thought the world of him, looking forward to his visits and chatting non-stop from when he entered the house til leaving an hour or two later.

The day after Joanne's Christening when we were back visiting her at the hospital, we were asked if we could hang around to speak with one of the other surgeons who had been visiting a patient of his near Joanne's incubator the previous day as he was interested in speaking with us. Mr Peter Raine normally specialised on "burns" patients, but he wanted to speak with us about Joanne.

After his ward round that day, he asked if we could follow him along to his office. There he detailed again Joanne's problems. He spoke kindly but rather negatively, so we were shocked when at the end he said he was willing to try to perform the "Kasai" operation on Joanne, so called after the surgeon who pioneered it in Japan. This operation involves joining up the bile ducts from the liver to the bowel. He re-iterated that they had never had any success previously in Scotland but said there were children living in other parts of the world who had benefitted from this procedure and that he felt that Joanne "deserved a chance". Three simple words. How awesome that one person could change the whole course of our lives with these words. How lucky are we to have medical people who on a daily basis are willing to go that extra mile for sick and needy people. Here was this man who had the power to change everything. A quiet unassuming man in his early 40s. Our hero!

I believe that surgeons and medics like Mr Raine are not appreciated nearly enough, except of course when you are in a life or death situation, but their daily routine is one of extreme stress from start to finish and they always have to be on point with every decision they make. We should all consider ourselves extremely fortunate that there are still some people in the world with their kind of work ethic, and should not be so ready to take inappropriate action when things don't work out. After all, medicine is not an exact science, some people can't tolerate certain medicines, some treatments work on one person and not the other, operations don't always necessarily work out or cure the patient, so why are we so ready to blame doctors. In the main, and throughout our experiences in different hospitals over the years, these people do their very best to treat people with respect and to the best of their ability. But it is human nature that sometimes people make mistakes, and it is a fact that medics can't cure all, they are still learning, and there is still a lot of research to be done, so we need to accept all of that.

It is an awful responsibility for such people. The responsibility of changing people's lives. No guarantees given and no guarantees needed – just the courage to take the chance is all that some families want and need to give a little ray of light for a loved one who is without hope. There are many surgeons like Mr Raine in this country. And there are many doctors and nurses who work side by side, performing miracles every day either by improving lives or saving lives. It is the most underrated profession, but in my experience such people are not looking for any kind of glory. They just know that what they do is worthwhile and wish that they had more funding to enable them to do more. It would also be nice if they were appreciated more at times, because they do work under extremely difficult circumstances.

So, Mr Raine said he would leave Joanne a few more days to recover from what she had already gone through, and look at doing the operation as soon as possible after that. In the meantime, I was able to move back into the hospital to look after her.

Despite being told not to be too optimistic, we were absolutely euphoric on the drive home that night! Before we knew the prognosis, it would have been unthinkable that we would be so happy that our tiny baby daughter was to go through such intricate life changing surgery, but here we were thinking for the first time that, like the other parents on the ward, we did in fact have hope.

It seemed to me that it didn't matter if your child is sick or well, as a mother your instinct is the same - to look after that child. I could only treat her as any mother would their child. I was there to look after her, feed her, change her, talk to her, love her. Everything seemed so normal when it was just the two of us. She didn't look desperately ill. She wasn't in any pain. She was perfectly happy just being looked after and being fed. It was so hard to believe that this tiny baby was so ill. But here I was, on the morning of her op., washing my tiny baby – preparing her for an operation that would change her life in a way that was not deemed possible by medical professionals.

The operation went better than could ever be imagined and Joanne's recovery was so good that we were allowed to take her home to live as a family for the first time since she was born. Not, however, before being reminded by Mr Raine that Joanne was not "cured" and he was not sure whether or not she would benefit from the Kasai operation.

Coming home from the hospital for the first time with our baby was joyous of course, but filled with trepidation about the future. We had been living in a routine of hospital visits, hospital stays, sleepless nights and not eating properly while trying to be "normal".

Her nursery was prepared at home but needless to say Joanne slept in our room in her cot next to our bed. I was the one who got up most nights to feed her as John was working long hours in his job at the school. She wasn't a great eater. Slow to feed, but as Mr Raine had warned us that this might be the case, I was determined to ensure that she got all the nourishment she needed. You see, after the operation, they weren't sure what follow-on treatment would be needed, so the only prescription medications we were given were for vitamin supplements. They felt sure that Joanne would never get the nourishment she needed because of her liver problem, that she would never walk nor talk and that she could have brain damage. Mr Raine, although he was delighted to see her doing so well, made a point of reminding us of this at every appointment during the first couple of years after her operation. He also made a point of outlining the symptoms of her decline – what to look out for and pretty much telling us how she would die. He said if it got too much, then he would admit her back into hospital where they would provide nursing care at the end of her life.

During these appointments I would listen, but inside would be telling myself "that won't happen – I'll make sure it doesn't". I never felt it was arrogance that was driving me to this conclusion, I just knew that if anyone could prove him wrong, it would be Joanne.

When she was coming up to around 16 months old, although she was thriving as normally would be expected, she was still not able to walk on her own. I wasn't thinking that she would never walk, as the doctor had predicted. I wasn't concerned that she was a late starter. She had been running around with the help of a baby-walker for a while, but she just didn't seem to have the strength to stand and walk on her own. We had to find a way to help her find that strength.

We had never been complacent, always looking into research being carried out, looking for new treatments or procedures that could help prolong Joanne's life beyond what we were told to expect. We contacted hospitals in England, where we knew most young children with liver disease were treated, but they didn't carry out transplants on children at that time as they were still at the "experimental stage". Generally speaking, doctors here in the UK were very much against carrying out experimental treatments on children. (we learned later that they had carried out one or two liver transplants in England in young children but without success). We knew that liver transplants in children were being carried out in America, and had been in touch with a hospital in Boston about Joanne but because of Joanne's complications, they were not able to offer even a glimmer of hope. We were running out of time if we were going by the prognosis of 2 years maximum life expectancy that the doctors had given. To me, she was doing better than I could ever have hoped so it was hard to acknowledge the fact that this could all go so badly wrong and quite soon into the bargain. Ignoring all the negativity, and trying not to look too far ahead, it was still my goal that she would lead a normal life, so we had to find a way to get her walking on her own. John came up with the idea of trying homeopathy treatment, and so we got in touch with Mr Coutts – a homeopathic practitioner in Glasgow. We took Joanne along to see him, and he was very interested in her medical prognosis and history. However, he didn't want to commit to treating her without further research, so said he would contact us soon. After a two week wait, we were delighted to hear from him that he had consulted with other homeopaths in Glasgow and that they had all contributed their thoughts and agreed on a specific treatment that they felt would benefit Joanne. He posted out the medicine to our home, and refused to take any money for her treatment. All he asked was that we give it a try and keep in touch with him about her progress. We spoke to Mr Raine at the hospital, and he was happy for us to give Joanne the homeopathic medicine provided it did not do her any harm - as he said, there was nothing more they could offer by way of any treatments for her.

So we started on this course of homeopathic treatment, and within a couple of weeks Joanne was running around the house all by herself. I have no idea what the pills were meant to do, but she seemed to have lots more energy. Also, by this time she was of course chatting away like a budgie. And there certainly wasn't any sign of brain damage. Life was good.

We had plenty of visitors to the house and Joanne had lots of friends her own age to play with so she became very sociable too. She loved music – she had gotten used to it as I had the radio on every morning while busying around doing the household chores. Even as a very small baby she was used to listening to music, and sometimes I caught her trying to sing along in her baby-like fashion when she was sitting up in her pram (learning the words to songs word for word would come later). We usually ended up with me dancing around the livingroom and Joanne in my arms to some of our favourites.

3

Not long after Joanne's 2nd birthday, she started to deteriorate. Like all parents of chronically sick children, we had our endless visits to hospital for check-ups, and doctors when things weren't quite right, but when we were faced with what we had been dreading, we were totally devastated that Joanne appeared more jaundiced and was gradually becoming more unwell. John called the doctor out on the Sunday morning before Christmas, and as she couldn't detect any infection as being the cause, she concluded that it could be the beginning of the end for Joanne. We spoke to Mr Raine the next day, and he suggested we take her to the hospital for end of life care, as there was no treatment that they could give her to make her better. I was devastated, but declined his offer, and said I would nurse Joanne at home.

Christmas day was as good as we could make it under the circumstances. We had all her new presents lying underneath the Christmas tree (and beyond), and by the time she had opened them all with our help, you couldn't move in our living room for toys. Thinking back, I suppose we did try to cram everything in just in case the worst did happen, so she was a bit more spoiled than she would have been if she had not been so sick. But who doesn't spoil their children? We all do it. So she had a shedload of toys, and like most children her age, she was really only interested in one or two things that caught her eye and of course the wrapping and boxes that the presents came in. The toys came in handy anyway when we had our play time visitors. My friends Liz and Kay came regularly with their daughters, Gemma and Jacqueline and the three girls became great friends and played well together. There was no question of them fighting over a toy – there were loads to choose from. And at that time, Joanne was not getting out much, in fact she didn't get out at all for almost three months. She was badly jaundiced, she itched constantly and she was really unwell. The medics had nothing to offer in the way of conventional treatment. So once again, we turned to the homeopath. We had been keeping in regular contact with Mr Coutts anyway – visiting him at his Glasgow clinic with Joanne to let him see her progress and he had been keeping us supplied with her homeopathic medication free of charge. He was just so delighted that he was able to help, so when we told him about Joanne's deterioration, he asked for some time again to speak with other homeopathic doctors before getting back to us. We were not in a position to refuse him the time he needed, but we were desperately in need of immediate help for her.

I was nursing Joanne round the clock. She seemed to be in so much discomfort so sometimes I would be giving her a bath in the middle of the night, just to ease the itch she had from the build-up of bilirubin in her body. At other times I would be up all night trying to feed her just to ensure that she was getting enough nutrition as her appetite was so poor at this time. But most of the time she was lying in my arms, with me constantly scratching her body, her head, feet and arms, just to relieve the itch and allow her to get some peace. That seemed to relieve her discomfort.

I still remember one afternoon looking out of our front room window. I could just see far enough along our street to the turn that took you onto the road that led to shopping centre. A short walk to the shops - one I had taken frequently with Joanne in her pram or buggy. At that moment I remember thinking that I wished for nothing more than to take that walk together again round that corner. It seemed so long ago since we had been out. That was my new goal. Imagine that your only wish is taking your baby in her buggy and turning that corner. A Simple thing to most maybe, but we had a mountain to climb before that would happen. But, you know what? It was going to happen – I just knew it would.

Shortly after our conversation with Mr Coutts, he once again came to the rescue with a homeopathic remedy to hopefully help Joanne. At the time, it seemed our only hope. That, and the will of God. All we could do was hope and pray.

Looking after a sick child is difficult and draining. The stress involved is considerable. The whole family feels the pain, but mums and dads feel the guilt, anger and sheer exhaustion. You must face the many challenges head-on because you simply can't choose to opt out. You feel like a machine – you just keep going. I never had a proper night's sleep for the first seven years of Joanne's life, and only then because my doctor prescribed some sleeping pills to help me get into a better sleeping pattern. The first one I took knocked me out for hours, so I ditched them after that. There was no way I wanted to be out of it if my daughter needed me.

In our case, there were never any support groups that some parents may have had access to, simply because Joanne's illness was so rare and crudely put, terminal. So it seemed to me, that we and parents like us who had babies who were terminally ill, were just left to get on with things. Would I have wanted to attend if there was such a group? Would I have been able to listen to others in the same position as ourselves who had no future to look forward to with their babies? Probably not. Luckily for me, I think, was the fact that I wanted to look after my baby myself. I felt capable, and was more than willing to take on the job. It was inconceivable to think that anyone else would take on my role, because as a mother I believe it is inbuilt and instinctive to take care of your children and especially so when they are so very ill. In any case, Joanne's illness was a family issue, not just Joanne's issue, so we would get through it together.

Over the next few weeks, our lives were on hold. The only priority was to make Joanne as comfortable as we could and hopefully well again. It was a particularly trying time – waiting for things to get better - and with no foregone conclusion although it was clear to us that the medical professionals thought that the only outcome would be our baby's passing.

But Joanne's symptoms gradually began to subside. She became stronger and less jaundiced. So when Joanne was well enough our first trip out was a visit to the maternity hospital where she was born to visit my sister in law who had just given birth to a baby girl. It was now mid-March, and I began to look forward to the future. Not too far into the future, but day to day we began to do normal things again.

On a visit to the hospital in April, Mr Raine was a bit surprised to say the least to see that Joanne seemed to be getting back to her old self. He decided that he wanted to take some tests, something he had never done since her operation when she was just nine weeks old. He had always felt that it was not necessary to put Joanne through that, as he didn't have any expectations of the results being good. So when he got the results back he couldn't wait to phone us at home to tell us that they surprisingly showed that her liver function was much the same as it was when she had the operation. So, although there was damage to her liver, it had happened before her operation and there had been no deterioration since.

He talked about the "future" for the first time, and advised that I should enrol Joanne in a nursery so that she could get used to being away from me and mixing with other children and adults as it could be that she might have to spend times in and out of hospital in the future. It was fair to say that Joanne and I were like joined at the hip so I suppose he was right in subtly saying that we maybe should spend some time apart – all part of her development! For the first time ever he referred to her condition as "life threatening" instead of "terminal". I picked up on this right away. It was a big deal. It meant the world of difference in my opinion. I was secretly on cloud nine!

It is hard to remember all my thoughts that went through my mind as a mum with a chronically sick child. Motherhood is the hardest and most challenging job for any new mum anyway. You are overwhelmed with feelings of love and happiness. True and unconditional love, and you know that your child fully depends on you for EVERYTHING so you strive then to make everything perfect. But things are not always perfect, are they?

Here I was with a 2 ½ year old who wasn't meant to be here. It saddened me that my daughter was going to go through difficulties that I wouldn't wish on anyone. At that age though, I was grateful for the fact that she didn't know what lay ahead – she didn't know she was sick. We, her parents, would carry that burden and shield her from the harsh reality - for a while anyway.

Guilt seems to be a natural feeling that all mums have, whether it is because they feel they are not doing things right, aren't doing enough or because they have to go to work, and most mums will relate to this. It is an overwhelming feeling I have carried throughout Joanne's life and since her passing. But my guilt stemmed from the awful suffering my daughter had to bear as a baby and young child, and would have to face in the future. No-one could ever help me to overcome this feeling of guilt. I had carried this baby and given birth to her. Everyone who knew me well knew that I had done everything right during my pregnancy. I had already had a miscarriage the year before Joanne was born, even although I had stopped smoking, I never touched alcohol and I ate well throughout my pregnancy. So I had been even more careful to take it easy as well during my second pregnancy and not overdo things. Despite doctors telling me that Joanne's condition was not my fault, it was crippling to see this tiny person develop - even then she had an amazing personality - knowing that her future was so bleak. I would have done anything to change places with her. It was also so hard to see doctors and nurses look at Joanne in awe or sometimes pity, not really knowing how to react or the right things to say because they had no idea how she had survived so long nor how much longer she would live.

At this point, I had to change my way of thinking. No longer just a fight for survival. Joanne had proved that she could win that battle. She had done it once and she would do it again. Now I had to consider other things in life that were important to children growing up. Looking at her then, she was no longer a child with a multitude of problems - she was now a little bundle of hope. I had to believe that. I did believe that. Yes there would still be hospital visits. Yes, I would still constantly check to see if she was breathing while asleep in her cot. And yes, there would be good days and bad days, the good days being we go out places, we see new things, we visit people and enjoy life, and bad days we stay in, away from the germs and dangers of the outside world, and wait for things to get better – and pray.

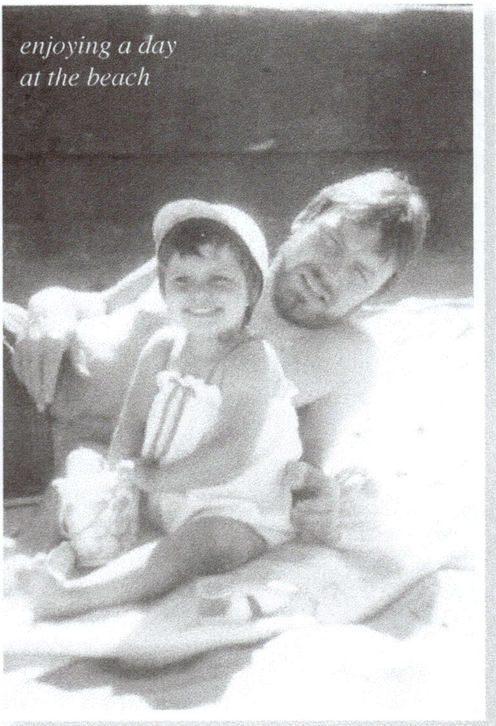

enjoying a day at the beach

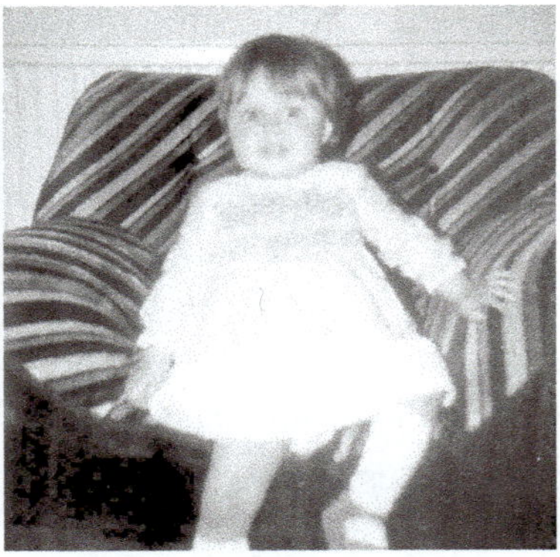

I can walk by myself now - just having a wee rest

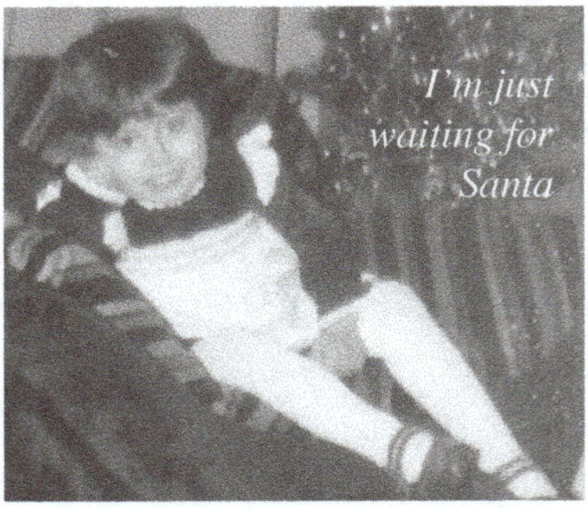

I'm just waiting for Santa

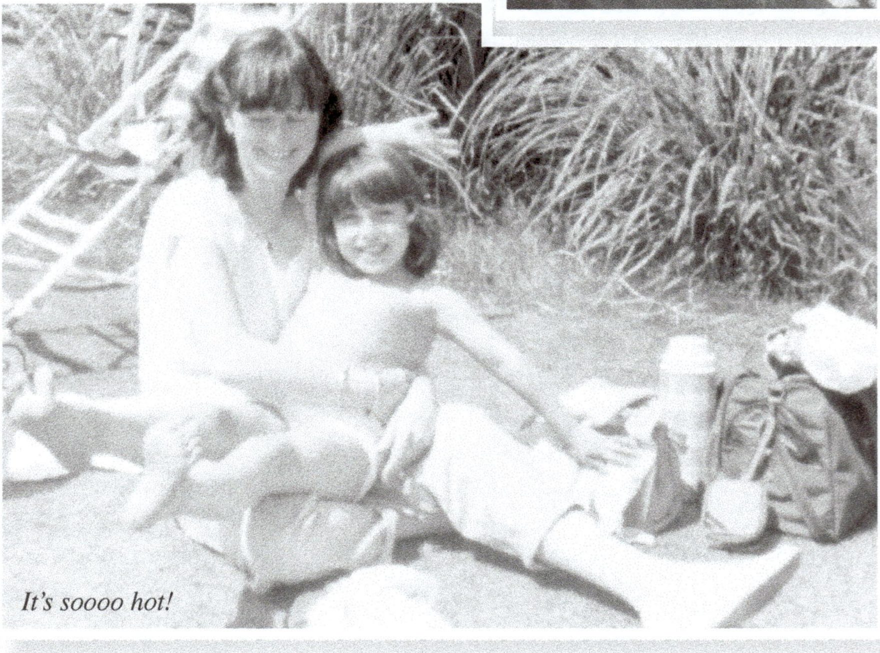

It's soooo hot!

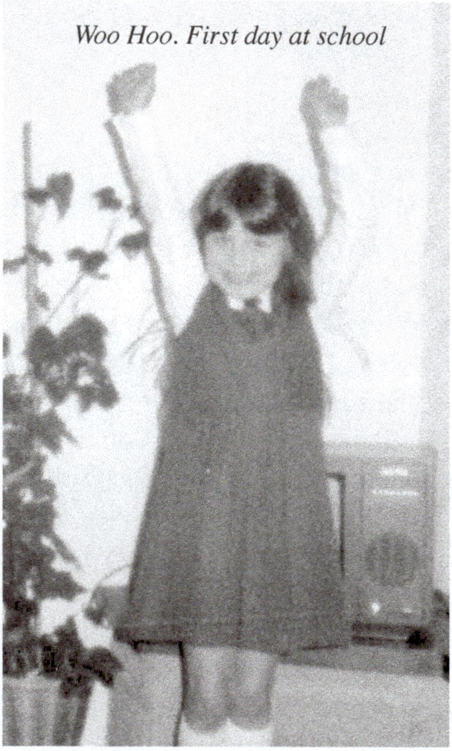

Woo Hoo. First day at school

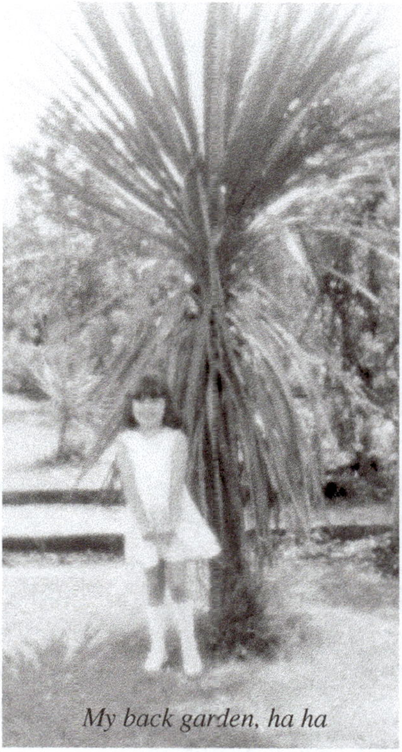

My back garden, ha ha

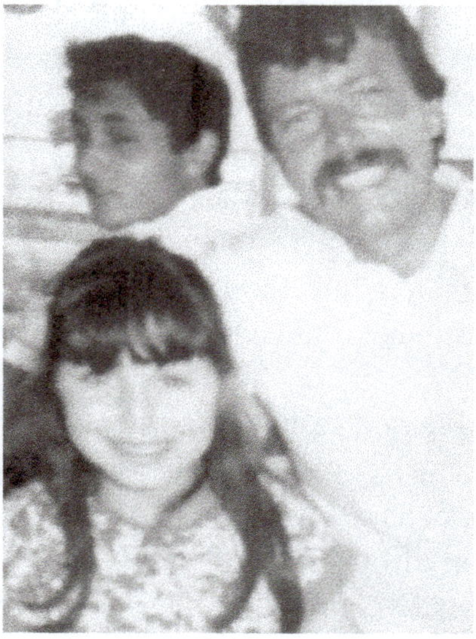

Loving my sunshine holiday

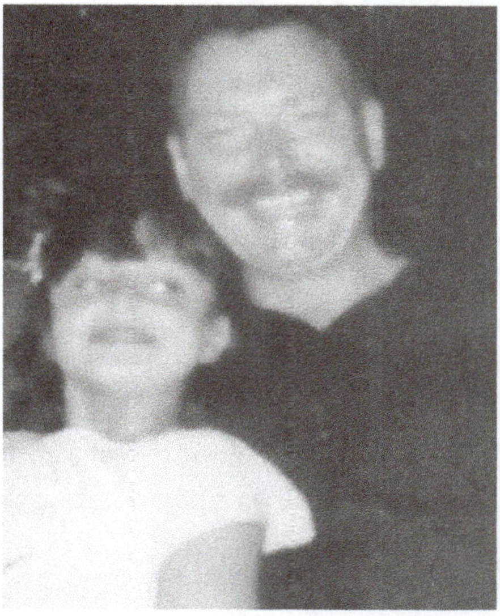

Another sunny holiday!

4

Being a mum to a sick child means that you see a side of life that you never knew existed, nor thought much about before. Your life revolves around doctors' appointments and hospital visits. You watch other mums in hospital waiting rooms with their obviously sick and fragile children. So many illnesses. You see their worry and their pain – written in their faces. I mean you REALLY see them. Because you have a better understanding of what their lives are like. It means that you constantly worry. You cry a lot and you rarely sleep. You try hard to do better – sometimes you win and sometimes you lose. You cry some more, and then you pick yourself up and start all over again. It's a never ending circle but you learn to accept the life you have been given. You get on with it. It would be a lot easier if you were certain that there was light at the end of the tunnel, but you don't have that luxury. And you get little or no encouragement from doctors that things will be ok. You live a day at a time. So that was our motto. One day at a time.

Things that used to seem important now just don't matter. Your whole world revolves around that sick child while everyone else's life moves on. It can be a very lonely existence. You feel isolated. Most of your friends have never experienced this and so don't really understand. Everyone now knows you as Joanne's mum. Even your oldest friends! Your conversations are about Joanne. Because you don't have a life of your own! But that's ok. In fact, that's great. There is nothing that mums like more than to talk about their children, whether they are sick or not! That's just what mums do. So in a lot of respects, you are just a normal mum.

My Joanne was a Godsend. I am blessed to have had her in my life, and to be her mum was an honour. I could honestly say that I could not ever have had a better child, even if I was allowed to hand-pick one. She gave me a purpose in my life. And ironically I could never have coped with the life I had been given without her. Because she had the courage of a lion. She was such a beautiful, sensitive, happy soul with a strong character, and so strong - it would have been impossible to give up on her through any of the difficult times we had to go through. But you have to balance your lives, you can't ever dwell on the negative aspect of any illness, and so I had to focus more on Joanne living her life, and less on fighting her illness.

So I would have to organise that nursery place that I never thought she would need. And I could actually daydream about going on holiday, something we were always told we couldn't do. It was as if we had been given the green light to live (more) normal lives – the world had opened up to us and we were going to enjoy it.

So Joanne started nursery school in the autumn that year. It was a tearful time for both of us. Every day was like " groundhog day" with Joanne in tears before we left the house and crying during the journey to her nursery school – she didn't want to go - and me in tears after I left her there. But the head teacher insisted that I persevere, and after a couple of weeks she settled and soon became the first to welcome any newcomers and comfort any of the other children when they were upset. Her nursery school teacher always greeted me with a smile after the initial upset, as she said Joanne just made her day. She was so chatty and to be honest, most adults loved her company.

She also joined the Sunday school at the church where Mr MacFarlane preached, and I became a Sunday School Teacher at the same time. The Superintendent, May Thompson, had suggested that I shouldn't teach Joanne's group, and that was fine with both of us. This continued right up until Joanne had to have her first transplant and throughout this time May and I became good friends. Although we only met from time to time afterwards, I always knew that I could rely on May if I needed any help. She was a kind, helpful soul, and was still there for me when Joanne was last ill.

Joanne's condition was stable during this pre-school age, and so John and I had discussed doing some charity work to help fund research into liver disease in children. Here we were, almost four years after Joanne was born and it seemed there had been little change regarding the possibility of any major advances on the management of biliary atresia. Research was not progressing as well as we would have hoped and liver transplants in children in Britain was still a taboo subject. There had been some publicity around a small child in England named

Ben Hardwick who had a liver transplant in Addenbrookes Hospital in Cambridge, but as he passed away shortly after due to complications, any plans of establishing a transplant programme for children were put on hold.

We knew we were on borrowed time with Joanne, but it seemed that the best we could hope for was for that borrowed time to continue. We knew that Joanne was not cured, and that any chance of a full recovery from her liver disease remained poor through lack of knowledge, so we decided to make our own contribution to research through fundraising.

John was still working as a school janitor at the time, and organised with colleagues throughout the area to take part in a sponsored walk covering a 20 mile route from Alexandria through Arden, Helensburgh, Cardross and Renton. The 11 janitors held sponsorship forms in each of their respective schools, and the response from children and parents was overwhelming. There were many supporters out on the day of the hike - mostly the school children and their parents who came out to cheer on their "jannie". It was a really enjoyable day, and made us realise that fundraising was fun! The event attracted the attention of the local newspapers, and this in turn attracted a lot of interest from the public.

We were amazed when the donations for the sponsored walk began to come in as we raised around £3000. The money was paid to the Michael McGough Foundation which was the main channel for fundraising for the research into liver disease in children. Michael was a six year old boy from Nottingham who had a liver transplant in America in 1979 – around the time Joanne was born. It was a pioneering operation at the time as the operation is entirely different to that carried out in adults and is also more difficult. Liver transplants had been carried out in adults for around ten years with promising results. However, Michael survived only a few weeks. Despite that, his parents set up the Foundation in his memory, working closely with the medical teams in Kings College Hospital in London where most of the research in Britain was carried out at the time, and still is today.

Not long after his family had returned from America I read an article in "The Sunday Post" about Michael. His parents had lived with Michael's illness for six years, and had been through all the hoops to get him to America, against the wishes of the doctors in England. Michael had been looked after by doctors at Kings College Hospital in London which was the centre of excellence in the whole of the United Kingdom for children with liver disease but when they had refused to carry out a transplant, Peter and Sonya McGough took their son to America for the procedure. At that time the operation was considered successful if the patient survived six months, but unfortunately, Michael did not. We contacted the hospital in America, but although they were very sympathetic, they were not able to offer any hope of Joanne ever getting the operation due to her complications.

So, we were very happy to help raise money for this charity, as it was all set up professionally with the right medical and other professional bodies on the board. All we could hope for was that things could progress in the UK and at some point in the future our daughter would get the help she badly needed.

It was 1983 when we started our campaign to raise money, and the amount we had raised from the sponsored walk was a huge sum in those days. But things didn't end there. Joanne was still at nursery school in Bonhill, and her head teacher, Mrs Russell, approached us to say that she would like to organise a Daffodil Tea with a prize raffle. Of course we were delighted, and on the day it raised the sum of £700. Again, a phenomenal sum of money even by today's standards. The event was well attended, and the raffle was drawn by a local professional footballer, Murdo MacLeod, whose daughter attended the nursery too. Murdo played for Glasgow Celtic football team, and he was able to offer us an autographed football to be signed by his Parkhead colleagues for a future raffle.

Money began to pour in from different events which people had organised throughout the area without our knowledge. A lot of the local school children wanted to help raise money. Children from St Martin's Primary School in Renton donated money when they sacrificed their pocket money during Lent, Alexandria Brownies held a daffodil tea and presented the proceeds to us at a Mad Hatters Tea Party, St. Ronan's Primary School held a collection, Levenvale School held a collection, and other school events included a summer fayre at Christie Park Primary School.

We also received money from a local pub's social club, a donation from TGWU, a keep-fit class who carried out a sponsored walk, a hypnotist show, local businesses, and numerous sponsored events carried out by friends and people we didn't know or hadn't seen since our school days! And a road sweeper who found a £5 note while he was doing his work along the main street, handed into the police. When it wasn't claimed, he got the money back, but instead of keeping it he decided to give it to the fund. We were overwhelmed by how things snowballed and by the generosity of local people.

We were approached by a Cash and Carry firm who often donated money that they raised at their annual staff dance to a charity. Margaret Diamond, the member of staff who normally organised these events, lived locally, and had put our name forward to be the recipients this time round. She told us she cried when she read Joanne's story in the local paper, and went straight to her boss with the idea of raising money for research into liver disease in children. They decided to make it a public event and were hoping for support from local people. Mrs Diamond truly was a diamond. She put her heart and soul into organising this event, and was able to get all the food for free, musicians for free, and booked the local newly-built Burgh Hall for free. She also managed to get a mountain of prizes, donated by businesses who used the Cash and Carry.

On the night, most of the local dignitaries attended the event. Almost half of the evening was dedicated to a race night – a fairly new idea at the time – as Margaret had found this to be a good fund raiser in the past. £2312.00 was raised. Typically they had raised around £1000 at these events, so this was a record amount so far for them.

Every week people were handing in money to John at the school or posting money to us at home. Complete strangers were doing whatever they could, donating whatever they could afford.

We agreed that we couldn't go on asking people to give over and over again. We also didn't want too much attention or the spotlight on Joanne as she was nearing the age of going to Primary School herself, so we decided to organise our final event. We had achieved so much so far by doing so little. But I am sure it was Joanne's gorgeous pictures that stuck in the minds of people who read her story in the local paper. She was such a happy smiley little girl, and that never changed.

So our final event was to be an afternoon disco in the local leisure centre, something for the children to enjoy – something to give back for all the support we had received. Needless to say, the event grew arms and legs.

John's sister, Agnes, got in touch with Radio Clyde radio station, and before we knew it one of their well-known DJs, Bill Smith – offered on air to come to the event and bring with him a load of freebies for the children and prizes for a raffle. We literally took over the whole of the leisure centre that day. In one area we had the children's disco, in another we had a coffee afternoon going on for the mums and dads, and in another hall we had around a dozen stalls including baking, jewellery, knitting, etc., with a huge tombola on the stage, and a raffle stall just beside it. We had so many prizes we were giving them out two at a time. The event was an overwhelming success, and just a perfect way to round off our fundraising activities. In eleven weeks we had raised over £12,000.00 with the help and generosity of people in our local community. It is still a lot of money by today's standards, but back then it was quite something.

Even the charity itself wanted us to run a "Scottish Branch" as we were doing so well, and were disappointed when we had to turn them down. We told them that we would maybe do an annual event in future, but we felt that the local people had shown enough support in the meantime.

It wasn't the end of fundraising for me though, as shortly after we had made this decision I was visited by Dr Elizabeth Scott, a local GP. I wasn't one of her patients, but she was impressed by the amount of money we had raised, and asked me to join her committee of fundraisers. She was involved in a number of charities, but her main one was to raise money for research into all child illnesses, including liver disease. How could I refuse? I had caught the bug. I enjoyed being involved in the events we held and found that it was a distraction for me, away from the worries of Joanne's illness. I can honestly say I probably wouldn't have got so involved in charity work had it not been for Joanne. Just one more way she enriched my life.

5

On the face of things, we were living a perfectly normal life. We had our child who was growing up in a happy environment, doing normal things and enjoying her life. Joanne always loved listening to music, and her tastes were varied. One of her first "idols" was Shakin Stevens, so when she was four years old I took her to her first "gig" at Edinburgh Playhouse to see "Shakey". From then on there was no stopping her. It just became the norm for Joanne that if she saw a band or a singer on the TV or heard a song on the radio that she liked, she wanted to go and see them live and very often we did! She also developed a great sense of humour, so we visited the theatre a lot to see comedies or comedians that were doing the rounds in Scotland, such as The Steamie, Francie and Josie, Rab C Nesbit, Billy Connolly to name but a few. Generally after a show we would chat about it in the car on the way home. It always amazed me that Joanne could recite the sketches almost word for word afterwards. Nothing wrong with her brain then! She was exactly the same with songs. She knew the ones she liked off by heart after listening to them just once or twice. I know there are plenty of people who can do that, but my heart would burst with pride – especially since we were told in the beginning that she could have brain damage.

I have to say though, this only happened with music and theatre – the things she was interested in. To be honest, school work didn't really do it for her, and I used to joke with her that I wished she paid as much attention in school – she could have been a child genius!

Although Joanne attended a mainstream school, she missed quite a lot of her education because of her health issues, and really wasn't that bothered about catching up with what she had missed. And in all fairness to her, education was the least of our worries. She was doing ok, so we didn't put too much emphasis on her schooling. We were happy that she was fitting in well with her classmates, and seemed to enjoy going to school. Her dad was the janitor, and that worked well for us, because we got to hear what she was up to first hand from the teachers. One example was when her class teacher told John about an incident in the class that day. A boy who sat nearby Joanne in class had put his hand up to attract the teacher's attention. "Please Miss, Joanne's sleeping" he said. "Just leave her" the teacher replied. "But please Miss, she's snoring, and I can't concentrate on my sums". Teacher had to laugh at that one. The boy was never usually interested in his sums anyway. Another example was when another teacher asked John if it was necessary for her to be allowed out of class regularly to go to the toilet. Joanne had been doing this a lot the last day or two and the teacher just worried that she may have a wee problem that we weren't aware of. He assured her that Joanne didn't have any infections or other recent problems that meant she needed to go more than anyone else in the class and she could wait til playtime like the rest of her classmates, but he said he would speak to her about it anyway. Before he got the chance, he noticed Joanne wandering along the corridor shortly after his conversation with her teacher. Sure enough, she was heading for the toilets, so he followed her. When he popped his head round the door, there she was in full flow – gabbing to one of the workmen who was up on a ladder carrying out maintenance work. When he saw John he tried to explain that Joanne had been coming in "for a blether" the past couple of days, and he had been telling her that she would get into trouble and so she should get back to class, but Joanne just said, "it's all right – the teacher knows I am at the toilet". Not a care in the world.

Another time she came home from school with her best school friend, Gillian Grigor. They had been best pals since starting school and spent a lot of time together out of school too. They came running up the path, Joanne excitedly saying "mum, I know what to get you for your Christmas present". I held my breath, wondering what was coming next. Apparently there was a stray cat that had wandered into the school in the last week or so, and it seemed that all the children wanted to adopt it, including Joanne. "Dad said he would bring it home later for you to see it first, but it's a Christmas present from me". What was I supposed to say to that! When John got home later, he said there was a wee cat that had been hanging around the school, but it was a beautiful clean wee thing and it looked as though it was well cared for, so he was sure it belonged to someone. Joanne wouldn't let it go, and wanted us to find out if it was someone else's or not, so that she could take it home (for MY Christmas present). So we phoned the vet to see if he knew of anyone who had lost their cat (he wasn't aware of anyone), and we put an advert in the local paper in the "Lost and found" as well as asking around locally. In the meantime, it started "following" Joanne home from school each day. With no response to our notice in the newspaper or our other attempts to find the owner, we were now the proud owners of the school cat, which Joanne named Garfield.

Joanne was turning out to be quite the character, and had a way of getting what she wanted – in the nicest possible way. Although I did overhear her telling her friends "If I ask my mum for something and she says no then I just ask my dad and he always says ok". Typical of children her age, but usually parents are the last to know they are being played.

By his own admission, John didn't really have a really close relationship with Joanne until she started school where he worked as the janitor. He was always doing things to make life easier for me, and was very good at doing all the housework, cooking and ironing without even being asked as well as doing a bit of shopping when needed. In her pre-school years, it was true to say that Joanne and I spent most of her awake time together. We were often out visiting friends or at my mum's when she was well. Joanne also loved out shopping or out for lunch with me and my mum or friends.

But the main reason for not seeing much of her dad was that he worked long hours in the school. In those days the school building, which is over 100 years old, required a lot of updating. They still had an old fashioned heating system in play, meaning that John had to start work at 6 o'clock in the morning to get the boilers going to make sure that the school was warm enough for the children coming into school at 9 o'clock. It was also the time when he had to clean the playground areas and do his safety checks at the start of the day. He would often have a break when the children were all in class, and was able to spend some time with Joanne and I then, but usually doing more practical things like going to the shop for things like milk and bread rather than spending fun times together. He would often not get home until 10 or 11 at night as there were usually community classes going on most nights in the building after school. So normally during the week he only spent brief times at home throughout the day when he could get a break for lunch or a bite to eat at tea time before going out again to prepare the school for evening lets.

So when Joanne started school, I was the one left feeling a bit redundant. She wanted to stay behind in school when it came to home time, as that is when she spent a lot more time with her dad. She would go to his office after school had finished to have a wee blether with the cleaners who worked in the evening. They would make her a cuppa and a snack, and she would sit with them chatting away before they started their work. It was also this routine that introduced her to some of the maintenance workers, so she wasn't at all shy about chatting to them when they were working in the school (not always after school time but also when she should have been in class, as I mentioned earlier).

She was right at home in the school, it was easy for her to use it as a play area after school, and she often stayed behind with one or two of her friends. Running around in the assembly hall or "playing" the piano in the hall. Joanne was doing well at that time, and I seemed to have a lot of free time, so I had the idea of getting a job. I thought I would be able to do agency work, which would give me the opportunity to work hours that suited me and I wouldn't be tied down to anything permanent. And so for the next couple of years I was able to work hours that we could work around. On occasions when Joanne was unwell, my mum was there to look after her which she was more than happy to do. When Joanne caught some of the usual childhood illnesses that were doing the rounds, like measles, chickenpox etc she often suffered more than most and it usually took her a wee while longer to get over it. But it didn't bother Joanne being a bit poorly, because she always bounced back and she rather enjoyed the time with her nana who pandered to her every need. My mum just loved her to bits, and her only grumble was watching videos such as "Annie" on repeat for days on end!

During these times when things were going well, we managed to get away on holidays, visiting places like Southport, Morecambe, Scarborough, Wales and the north of Scotland. We all enjoyed these holidays, and Joanne found it easy to make friends on our travels.

But of course, the weather was never predictable, and so we asked permission from Mr Raine to take Joanne abroad for a nice wee break in the sun. He cautiously agreed, provided that we didn't venture too far and were very careful with what she ate and drank. So at the age of six, Joanne had her first foreign holiday to Spain. We went in May, hoping that the climate wouldn't be too hot and exhausting. Everything went well, and so it became the first of many holidays abroad. We didn't venture further than Europe, though, and had many happy memories of relaxing, fun family holidays.

One holiday memory that sticks in my mind was when we went to Rimini in Italy. Joanne was around 8 years old, and we went in July that year with our friends, Liz and Monty and their daughter Gemma. I had known Liz since we were young, growing up as neighbours and friends. Joanne and Gemma we close since they were babies, and were more like cousins than friends. I remember we visited San Marino one very hot day, the temperature was over 120 degrees Fahrenheit, and we were wandering round a street market when Joanne had a nose bleed. One of the stallholders called us over, saying his daughter often suffered from nosebleeds in the extreme heat, and he wanted to help. So he sat beside Joanne and tipped her head back, maybe not the right thing to do, but he said it worked for his daughter. Joanne was trying to say something to him, but as he was Italian he couldn't understand her accent and he looked at me to interpret what she was saying. As I leaned forward to hear her better, she asked "who is that singing?" Being in the middle of market stalls, there was music blaring out of nearby speakers. The song was "Raspberry Beret" by Prince. People who know Joanne will know the significance of that day. The first day of Joanne's journey as No.1 Prince fan! Who else, I wondered, would be interested in the music blaring out of speakers when you are in the middle of a major nosebleed! When her nose eventually stopped bleeding, we couldn't leave the market until we found the music stall selling the Prince tapes .

Around this time, Joanne was a huge fan of River Phoenix, a young American actor, singer and as he got older he became quite political and vocal about the environment and changing the world. She first saw him in the iconic film "Stand by Me" and although I think he was her first "crush" she became interested in stories of his alternative type of upbringing. He was brought up by his parents in a commune of "hippies", and Joanne admired him because he wanted to break away from this lifestyle, he wanted to change the world, he was interested in the environmental issues and he believed in his ideals intensely. She had posters of him all over her bedroom walls as well as buying every book or magazine that had a story about him. She may not have been interested in academics, but from a young age she was very interested in the world we live in and the different lifestyles of people living in different parts of the world. I was a bit worried, though, that at 8 years old she had thoughts of replacing her bedroom posters of River Phoenix with posters of Prince.

6

I don't think there was an exact time when I noticed that Joanne's health was not as good as it had been. I think that it was a gradual thing - more that she was catching bugs and viruses more – and let's face it, what child doesn't pick up these nasties when they are at school. But with each of these common illnesses, her recovery was not so good and so her health didn't quite get back to where she had been before each bout of illness. She was still functioning ok and never complained but her colour wasn't so great, and her eyes had become more green. The whites of her eyes were never white anyway, and that was something that we had learned to live with. But they were no longer just slightly off colour – now the green tinge was becoming very dark. We still had our regular visits to the Sick Children's Hospital, and although her jaundice was becoming noticeable, nothing was done about it. This gradual decline probably went on for about a year or so with her catching infection after infection and not making a full recovery each time. I knew things were bad by the growing number of people who would stare at her when we were out shopping. They probably couldn't quite figure out what was wrong with her, but it was clear that she was not a healthy child. Even children in the school were asking her why her eyes were green, and some joked that she was a Ninja Turtle. This was very upsetting for me. I felt helpless, and wanted to scream at them all to just leave her alone.

One day when I came home from work Joanne was upstairs in my bed while John was waiting for me downstairs. He said that Joanne was complaining of pains in her legs in school, and was finding it difficult to walk. By the time he had got to her class to take her home she couldn't walk at all and he had carried her home. He had also phoned the hospital to speak to Mr Raine, and was told to take her to the hospital in the next few days if things didn't improve.

When I went upstairs to Joanne she had had a nap and was feeling better. She got up and was able to walk around with a bit of difficulty. But we went to the hospital after a couple of days as she still wasn't able to walk without pain. Mr Raine explained that he thought it was probably arthritis, a symptom of her liver disease. When this was confirmed, we were seen by another consultant, a specialist in this field, who took more tests to ensure that her body would be able to withstand medication he wanted to prescribe to alleviate the problem. When he was happy with the results of the tests, we were given a prescription to ease the pain and symptoms of the arthritis.

Joanne had taken only two of the tablets before she was taken home from school again feeling unwell. She said that she didn't feel sore, but thought she "had butterflies in her tummy" and was feeling strange. It was 8th June 1990 I remember, and the start of the World Cup tournament was showing on the TV. That evening, John was watching the football in the dining room while Joanne and I cosied up on the sofa in the lounge, settling in to watch a film. After a while Joanne said she felt sick. I went through to the kitchen to fetch a basin, and in the meantime I asked John to go sit with her. When I returned Joanne was sitting on her dad's knee and projectile vomited before I had a chance to reach her with the basin. However, as she continued to be sick into the basin, I noticed the dark colour of what we assumed was vomit. It was difficult to see with only the light of the dim lamps in the lounge. John actually asked if she had been drinking cola, but I knew it wasn't that – it was blood. Joanne was haemorrhaging. I ran to the phone and phoned for an emergency ambulance. I tried not to let Joanne see the panic in my face, and calmly told her that I just wanted to take her to the hospital to get her checked out. I had put on the outside lights and left the front door open as suggested by the assistant I had spoken to on the phone, but after what seemed like an age, with no sign of the ambulance, I decided to take Joanne to the hospital in the car. I put the basin on the floor at the back of the car, and after cleaning and changing her, I wrapped Joanne up in a blanket and drove to the hospital. I knew it was not the best thing to do, and I would probably get a telling off for doing so, but the hospital was literally on our doorstep, 2 minutes away by car and I was frantically worried that the ambulance might not get to us in time.

When we arrived at the hospital, I ran into the emergency room and showed one of the nurses the contents of the basin. I told her my daughter was in the car, and she had just vomited what I was showing her. Immediately she ran out to the car pressing an emergency button on her way, and was then followed by a few other colleagues who all took over the situation. Joanne was taken into the emergency room and was immediately put on drips and given oxygen to try to stabilise her. All the while I was by her side trying to comfort and support her.

We were there for some time when an ambulance crew arrived with another patient. I overheard one of the crew tell a nurse that they were leaving to pick up a 10 year old girl at our address. The nurse was able to tell them that she was already being attended to in the emergency room. She then came back in to tell me that on this occasion I had made the right decision to take Joanne to the hospital myself, as every minute counts in a situation like this.

We were there for hours before the staff decided that Joanne was stable enough to transfer her to the Sick Children's Hospital in Glasgow and so during the night she was transferred to the specialist hospital for further investigation and treatment. The first of many "blue light" ambulance journeys.

I travelled with Joanne in the ambulance. John, who had stayed at home to phone my brothers and his sister to give them the news, met us with our siblings at the Sick Children's Hospital. When we arrived in the ambulance, there was no bed available for Joanne, so we had to wait in a side room for one to become available. She was constantly monitored, but she wasn't seen by a specialist and wasn't given any treatment and it was several hours before she was actually taken onto a ward. Unknown to us, staff had been in touch with Mr Raine during the night, and he insisted that Joanne was to be given a bed on his ward. It was now Saturday morning, and as was his habit, Mr Raine arrived to do a ward round. He was visibly upset that this had happened, and although he was horrified, he also tried to justify giving Joanne the medication to treat the arthritis. They had, after all, carried out the appropriate tests and more to ensure that it would not harm her. Yet here we were – she had had a massive internal bleed and was very sick. This was a rare side effect with this medication, and there was nothing to indicate that it would affect Joanne this way, given the results of the various tests they had carried out before prescribing it - they had been especially cautious. She was still on oxygen and drips, and now it was a waiting game to see which way things would go.

It was not a speedy recovery, but day by day, I could see the old Joanne coming back to us. It was heartbreaking to watch our daughter in this situation. The poor wee soul was just 10 years old and didn't know what was going on. She was very weak, and it was some time before Mr Raine was able to carry out an exploratory operation to see where the bleed was actually coming from. Unfortunately, he was unable to find the source of the bleed, but was keeping Joanne in hospital, fearing that there could be a recurrence of the problem. I had moved in to be with her.

Joanne had been in hospital a couple of weeks, when a show we had booked was on at the Kings's Theatre in Glasgow. She had been asking me if we would be able to go, as she had been looking forward to it, but I knew Mr Raine was still seriously concerned about Joanne's condition and was reluctant to let her go, even for a few hours and even though she seemed a million times better than when she was first admitted to the hospital. Eventually he caved in – I think it was Joanne's wee petted lip – but with strict instructions that we went to the theatre and then straight back to the hospital. I phoned John with the news, and instructions on what clothes to bring for the outing. So that evening we went to see "The Steamie" at the King's, and it was just the medicine she needed. It seemed to do both of us the world of good, just getting out of the hospital environment for a while. It was just the boost Joanne needed, and it wasn't long after that that she was discharged. We were overjoyed to get her home, but the downside was that the day she was discharged, Paul and Linda McCartney turned up at the hospital unannounced, and gave an impromptu concert for the children and staff who could manage to go along. Being a massive Beatles fan, I was gutted I missed out.

We had a holiday booked to go to Portugal in September that year, but because Joanne had had such a hard time we booked a last minute week's holiday down in Torquay in July. They were having such beautiful weather down south at the time, and so we took off with my mum and a friend of Joanne's for a week of sun and relaxation.

After a few days of enjoying the sunshine, we noticed that Joanne seemed a bit lethargic. We didn't want to be complacent, so we asked the owner of our holiday apartment for the name of a GP. When we took Joanne along to see him, he did the usual checks but said that blood pressure etc. were all perfectly normal. We knew what to look for if she was bleeding, and none of that had presented. But she just didn't seem right. He thought it might be the extreme heat. He was, after all, sitting in his consulting room in shorts and polo shirt sipping a beer. Not the norm for any GP, is it? But the weather was unusually hot even for the south of England. So he gave us his private phone number, and said if we were still concerned about anything to give him a call and he would phone an ambulance to get Joanne into hospital.

Sure enough, later that afternoon, my mum noticed that Joanne's stool was black when she was at the toilet. So I immediately telephoned the GP and within minutes there was an ambulance outside our apartment to take us to Torbay hospital.

John and I went with Joanne in the ambulance, leaving my mum in the flat with Joanne's friend. After their initial assessment, Joanne was given a bed on the ward. They wanted to keep her in overnight just to be on the safe side. John left to go back to the flat and I waited with Joanne. She was the only patient on a 2 bed ward, so I was told I could use the other bed overnight provided it wasn't needed for a new admission.

Not long after John left, we were sitting chatting when Joanne said she felt sick. I didn't even get to fetch a sick bowl before she projectile vomited blood. I pressed the emergency button, and almost instantly there were four or five nurses surrounding us. One of them was trying to push me away, but I wouldn't budge. My daughter needed me there for reassurance and I wasn't stopping them from doing their job. I kept hold of her hands telling her she would be all right. Doctors arrived, and although she vomited up more blood, it wasn't nearly as bad as her first bleed at home.

The hospital staff were truly amazing. They couldn't have done any more than they did for us. When John arrived back later that evening, they had already been in touch with Kings College Hospital in London, and made arrangements for Joanne to be transferred there. They were also trying to arrange for the air ambulance to come and pick us up from the hospital to get her to London, and continually kept popping in to check on Joanne and update us with any progress. John and I agreed that he would drive back to Scotland with the others straight away, then make his way down to London the next day. It was

Friday 13th July, and the next day was my 39th birthday. Joanne was to be admitted to the high dependency unit at Kings College Hospital that night and be prepared for surgery first thing on Saturday morning.

It turned out that the RAF helicopter which was to take Joanne and I to London was still out at sea, and so they quickly arranged for an ambulance instead. The consultant on the ward travelled with us, and we were given a police escort all the way. Both the ambulance and police car had blue lights flashing all the way there. I can't remember how long it took, but the consultant said we averaged over 100 miles per hour!

7

We arrived at the hospital in the dead of night. Joanne's assigned nurse on the high dependency unit was waiting our arrival. She had a tough job that night. Joanne's heart rate kept dropping and she had to juggle her meds. to keep her stable. At 8 o'clock the next morning Joanne was wheeled down to the operating theatre, with me by her side. King's College Hospital is a very old building with very narrow corridors. The operating theatre was down in the basement, and the place reminded me more of a prison than a hospital. Mr Edwards, the surgeon, was all gowned up and waiting our arrival. He spoke briefly to me, telling me not to worry, and trying to put me at ease said "I've done this operation before". It didn't help. No mum wants to see their child so sick, nor go through this ordeal. I walked back to the ward in tears. Here I was in a strange hospital in God knows wherein London, and didn't know a soul. I got back to the ward, and started tidying round Joanne's bed for her return, giving me something to do to take my mind off things. One of the nurse's came over and took me to their staff kitchen to make me a cuppa.

We got chatting, and I soon realised that Joanne was in very capable hands. It was a difficult situation for me – I didn't know much about this hospital except that it was considered the centre of excellence for children with liver disease. But I didn't know any of the staff, didn't know their success rates, and just felt totally isolated. When you have this knowledge, it can be reassuring. But that nurse soon put me at ease. Mr Edwards was an excellent surgeon, she said, and Joanne would be fine in his capable hands. The nursing staff on that ward were in a different league too. Every child on the Mountbatten Ward was considered very seriously ill - some with cancer, some with heart problems, but most with liver disease. These very sick children were in the best place receiving the best treatment possible.

But it was obvious too, and concerning, that the hospital was seriously underfunded. There wasn't much cleaning going on for a start and it was clear that we parents were responsible for keeping our child's bed area clean and tidy. Joanne's bed was to the front next to the nurses' desk in an 8 bed space ward. Luckily so, as it turned out, as there were some mums at the end of the ward who didn't recognise the importance of ensuring that the environment was kept clean and free from infection. It wasn't unusual to hear the ward sister telling them off for leaving dirty nappies lying around among other things. But it seems crazy that our hospitals are being underfunded and when that happens, then services are cut. So usually that will mean less cleaning. Less cleaning may result in a greater risk of infection – and we all know how additional infections can affect people who are already sick. It is so important that the children get the best fighting chance to get well, so politicians need to wake up to the fact that our NHS needs more money – not less.

It was a beautiful sunny morning and the temperature was rising. Staff were allowed to work in their normal clothes for the first time ever as it was too hot to work in uniform. It was so hot that all the local shops had run out of fans. They had been bought up by staff and families of patients alike, and were everywhere you looked on the ward and throughout the hospital, and it still wasn't enough. After my morning cuppa, the nurse encouraged me to go out for a walk. It would be a while before Joanne was out of theatre, and I should get some fresh air. There were no mobile phones as such in those days – one very rich parent visiting the ward had a "brick" which was still a rarity then to have even that - so I decided to go out and look for a phone box to update John at home.

As I walked away from the hospital, I decided to take a left turn and found myself walking down a hill towards what seemed like a shopping area. Sure enough, I soon found myself in the thick of it and found a phone box, so was able to phone home to let John know that Joanne was in surgery and wouldn't be out for another couple of hours. John had made arrangements to travel down to London by train and would be leaving shortly.

So I spent the next while in a daze, just trying to pass time until I could get back and see that my daughter was ok. I walked back up the hill towards the hospital, but knowing that Joanne would still be in theatre, I continued walking further past the hospital and found myself going in to this beautiful park, which just sat immediately behind the hospital grounds. On a beautiful sunny day, with the birds chirping in the trees and children enjoying the paddling pool and play area in the park, it was so peaceful. Surely things would work out. It was my birthday for goodness sake. Surely nothing could go wrong on my birthday.

After a while, I made my way back to the hospital ward. The girl in the bed next to Joanne's empty bed was now awake, and her mum had come in to visit. Janine was around Joanne's age, and had biliary atresia. I learned over the next few days from her and her parents that Janine's health was good in comparison to Joanne. But she only had a mild form of biliary atresia to deal with, and it seemed that the Kasai operation she had when she was a baby had been a complete success. She lived in Surrey and was in for a regular check- up. I knew that there were different degrees of biliary atresia – and that Joanne's was severe – but it was also clear that Joanne's liver illness was seriously exacerbated by the other health problems she had.

I was waiting by her bedside when Joanne was eventually taken back onto the ward. She was on oxygen and lots of drips, but Mr Edwards said that he had managed to find and rectify the problem which caused her two haemorrhages. He was confident she would make a full recovery from the operation. She was fast asleep, so one of the nurses took me round to show me the parent accommodation near to the ward. There were cooking and washing facilities and sleeping accommodation for parents who did not live nearby. Since Joanne was expected to be in a while, we were offered a room. John arrived later that evening by which time Joanne was awake, although still a bit groggy.

The next few days passed with Joanne's condition improving every day. She became more aware of what was going on around her and was taking it all in. The consultant asked to speak to John and I one day and we were given an appointment for later in the day. He first of all explained what they had done to ensure that Joanne should not suffer from further bleeding. Then he went on to explain how ill our daughter was at this stage. Bluntly put, she needed a liver transplant, but the big question was, is she a suitable candidate for a transplant?

He told us they would like us to stay so that they could carry out a full assessment of Joanne's condition to see if it would be feasible. It was her only chance of survival. So there was nothing more to consider. We would, of course, stay in order that they carry out the necessary tests.

We left his office in a daze. I was terrified. A liver transplant in children was still relatively new, and the success rate was not great. Success was measured by the length of time the recipient survived i.,e, the operation was considered successful if the recipient survived a year after the operation (so it seemed that over time the life expectancy had increased from 6 months to a year) Organ transplants were not, and are still not, considered a cure. Despite this, I was kind of relieved that a transplant might now be an option. We thought at that time that there would be a cure someday or better management of her condition, so all we were hoping for by putting Joanne through this was buying her time until she would be able to live a near normal life with the support of medication.

When I went to phone home to let my family know I completely broke down. I had been trying so hard to hold it all together. I couldn't go back to Joanne's bedside and let her see me so upset. So it took some time trying to get myself together before I went back to join John and Joanne on the ward.

My two sisters in law, Lyn and Liz were arranging to come for a visit with Joanne's cousin Leigh, so having visitors was something for Joanne to look forward to. We were sitting chatting about this when Joanne started talking about one of the other patients who was in a side room along the corridor. She was 13 years old and had two transplants in a short space of time, both of which had failed. The doctors were refusing to give her a third transplant, and her mum was refusing to take her home. So there was a stand-off, with none of the staff able to discuss the situation, but everyone knew what was going on, and all the other parents expressing their thoughts and feelings on the subject. The family came from Wales after the girl had suffered liver failure caused by a virus at aged 12. Up until then she had been a perfectly normal healthy child. Mum busied herself each day at the hospital looking after her daughter, while dad stayed at home in Wales during the week to look after their other children, and visited the hospital at the weekend when he could arrange child care. Put yourself in those parents' shoes and I believe every single one of us would do the same.

Joanne had obviously picked up on what was going on, and was asking me about the girl's transplants. What did it mean? I tried to explain as best as I could. Joanne's reaction shook me - "Can I have one of them?"

Parents try to protect their children from all the bad things in life, and I had tried so hard to save my girl from worrying about her health and what might lie ahead. I was good at hiding my true feelings from her, and making her feel safe. Both John and I had got into the habit of NOT showing Joanne our true fears about her health, and so it was a shock to me to realise that she knew how ill she was.

But it gave me the opportunity to tell her that we would probably stay a while in the hospital so that they could check her out in case she did need a transplant at some point. We didn't know at this stage whether or not it was going to be possible anyway so it was best not to overload her with information. She had obviously had the stuffing knocked out of her and lost a lot of her confidence. If she was going to have major surgery, her head had to be in the right place. And so we carried on – making light of where we were and why, and being more positive in front of her than ever.

We had a few visitors down to London over the next few weeks while the hospital carried out their transplant assessment. Joanne was referred to Guys Hospital in London for assessment on her heart, as this was the main hospital in London at the time for cardiology patients, so we were relieved when we were told by the consultant there that he felt that Joanne's heart could withstand a transplant operation. We came home later in August, to await the decision of the medical team on whether or not Joanne would be a suitable candidate for a transplant. At this point, she was really poorly, spending most of her time in bed, and only getting up for a bath most days.

It was less than a week later when I answered the phone to a call from Kings Hospital. The junior doctor who had been given the task of phoning didn't have a very good bedside manner to put it politely. He was phoning to tell me that Joanne couldn't have a liver transplant, because the doctors felt she needed a new heart and lungs as well, and as that had only been carried out twice before without success, they were not going to offer this as an option. In fact, from some of the tests and scans they had taken, they were amazed that Joanne had survived this long. I asked how on earth they had come to the decision that she needed a triple transplant, since we were told by a heart consultant in Guys Hospital that her heart would withstand a liver transplant. He didn't have the answers to that and other questions I asked, so I asked him to get someone who did have the answers to call me back. The upshot was that Professor Mowatt phoned and asked us to come back down to London to discuss things face to face.

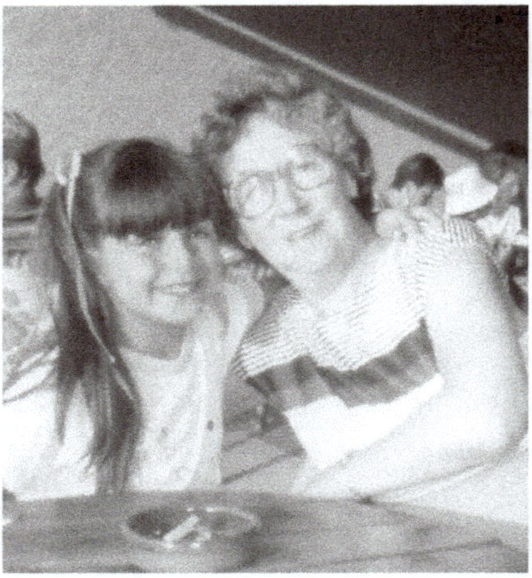

More sunny holidays

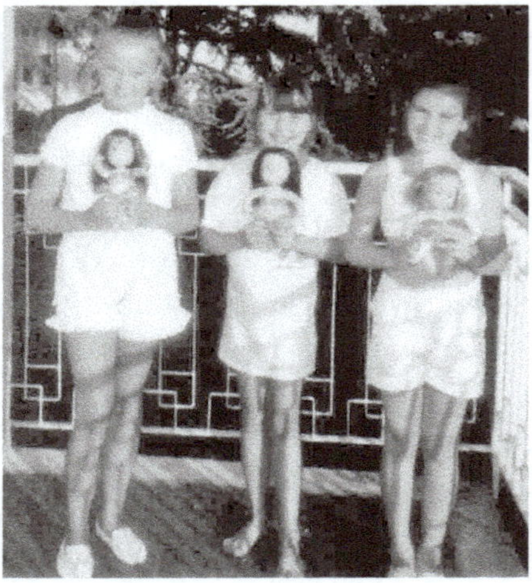

Holiday in Italy with Montagues

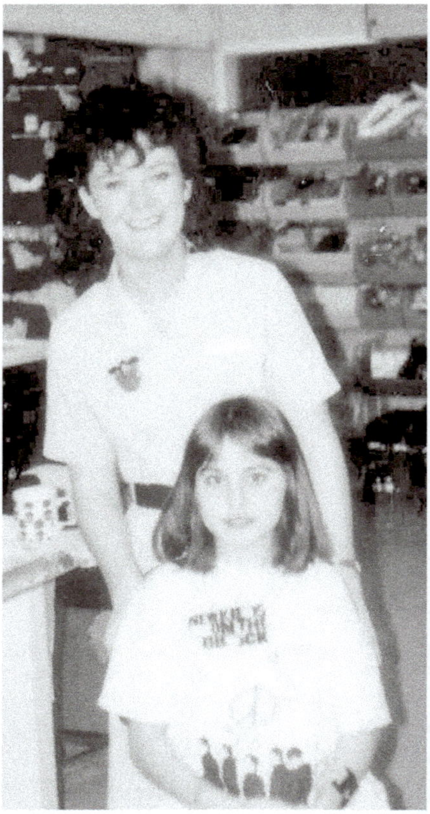

Leaving Addenbrookes after my transplants

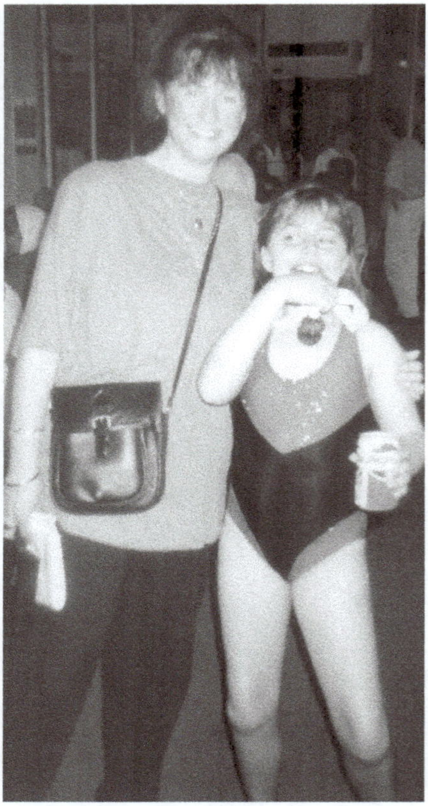

Winning silver medal for swimming at Transplant Games

Shakespeare Sisters

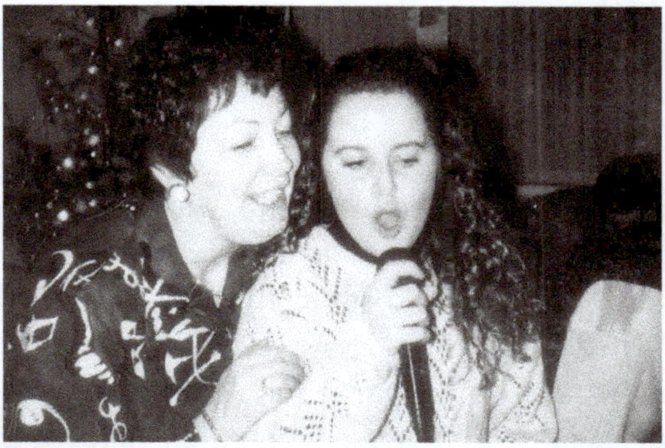

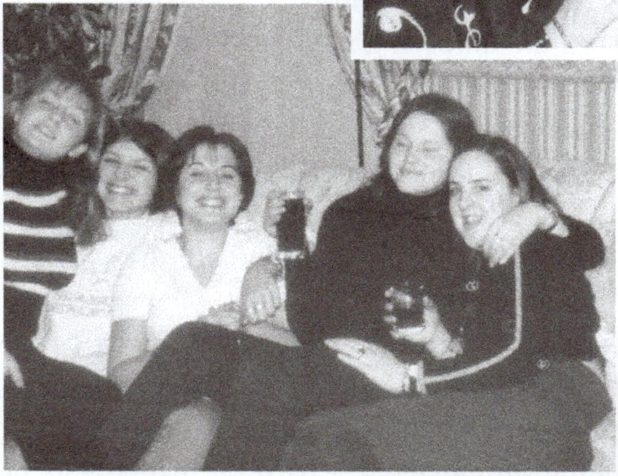

Girls on film

Blackpool with my friend Jaqueline

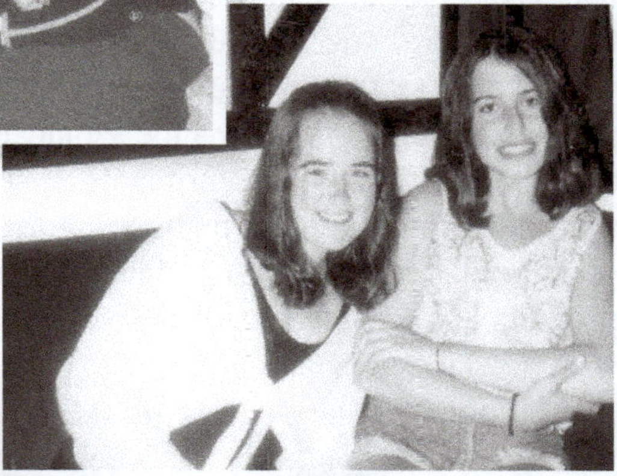

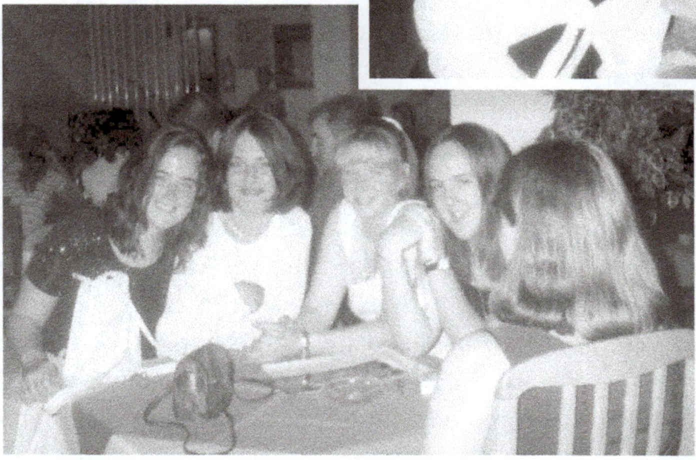

First holiday abroad with my girlfriends

8

It was August Bank Holiday Monday when we made our way down to London to meet with Professor Mowatt who had offered to come into the hospital specifically to meet us during the holiday weekend. When we arrived, Professor Mowatt went over the difficulties they anticipated with Joanne having such major surgery, and why they had decided not to put her through this knowing the outcome was bleak.

However, since my telephone conversation with the junior doctor, Professor Mowatt told us that he had discussed Joanne's case with colleagues at Addenbrookes Hospital in Cambridge, where they also carried out liver transplants in children, and colleagues in Papworth Hospital (which was in Peterborough at that time) where they carried out heart and lung transplants. The transplant team at Addenbrookes' had asked that he send down all of Joanne's notes and scans to the hospital there, and had also arranged transport for us to go there, anticipating that we would agree to speak to them too. The proposal, we were told, was that Joanne would have a triple transplant to be carried out by two different teams of surgeons – one doing the liver transplant and the other team doing the heart and lungs. This would probably be carried out at Addenbrookes in Cambridge. But before this could happen, we were to travel up to Cambridge that day to meet with the doctors in Cambridge

It is not what any parent wants to hear. Yes of course you want your child to be well, but the ordeal we were to consider putting our daughter through seemed a high price to pay.

I had been distraught when I thought my baby needed a liver transplant, so the feelings that a new heart and lungs were needed as well were just indescribable. I can remember that journey as if it were yesterday. It felt like we were going to the gallows. And there Joanne sat in the back of the car holding my hand, too sick to care.

When we arrived, we were taken to the admissions desk before being directed onto the ward where we were told someone would meet us. The hospital was a modern building and shining clean and bright and I remember a doctor in his white coat coming towards us as we entered the ward. "This must be Joanne – we've been waiting to see you" he greeted with a huge smile on his face. I asked where the loo was as Joanne needed to go to which he replied "excellent! Take this box and give me a sample while you are there!" He then took John round the corner where he said they had a bed ready for Joanne.

We didn't have a clue what was going on and we were totally unprepared. We thought we had just come down to London to speak with the consultant there, and here we were in Cambridge with Joanne being admitted onto the ward in a different hospital that we had no connection to.

Joanne and I came out of the toilet to look for John on the ward. I remember as we got closer to him I noticed he looked as though he had been crying. I was scared to ask, but when he told me the doctors had already looked at all of Joanne's notes, x rays and scans sent to them from Kings College Hospital, and they thought Joanne would only need a liver transplant - and wouldn't need a new heart or lungs. He said that, although it seemed as though she had a second heart murmur now and that her lungs were failing, they had found that these problems were as a result of liver failure, and were often rectified by giving a new liver. How the hell did they not say that in London! They obviously didn't know! God knows what would have happened if Professor Mowatt had not taken it upon himself to consult with doctors in another hospital. Another lesson learned. Get a second opinion. It was explained that Kings College Hospital in London was the lead hospital in liver diseases, but Addenbrookes Hospital in Cambridge was the lead hospital in liver transplants. Both hospitals were learning new things every day, but it seemed that they were not necessarily sharing what they were learning!

So John's tears were happy tears. Relief. A few weeks ago I was distraught when I was told Joanne needed a new liver, and now here I am ecstatic because I have been told she needs a new liver. Similar information – entirely different circumstances. But the best news – they are going to do it here in Cambridge.

The doctor who had welcomed us was named Steve Ravelle, and we were to call him Steve. Steve was from Rhodesia, and had worked in Harley Street in London as an anaesthetist (earning a shedload of money into the bargain) but had given it all up because he wanted to work with children. Steve was very posh and obviously well educated, but so down to earth and approachable. He was training to be a paediatric consultant, and along with Gabby Jamieson (a lovely German doctor who had settled in UK), they were the two doctors who ran the childrens' liver ward at the hospital.

The contrast between Kings College Hospital in London and this one was like night and day. This hospital was full of hope. The ward was clean and bright, and the staff was so welcoming. It was clear that this hospital was "flavour of the month" and was receiving plenty of funding. You learn a lot about how politics affects every aspect of our lives. For whatever political reason, Addenbrookes was getting all the NHS funding it wanted at that time, while King's College was struggling (a role that reversed through time, I learned).

As it was August Bank Holiday, and it is normal to try to get patients home in time for a holiday if they are well enough, the hospital was pretty quiet and was working on a skeleton staff that day. Steve explained that they wanted to carry out a few wee tests to add to Joanne's file, but they couldn't be done that day as they were really only able to deal with emergencies. We could go home when these had been done, and then it would then be a waiting game until a suitable organ became available.

At that time you are only thinking that your child has a chance to get well, so you block out any concerns you may have with organ transplantation. One thing you can't block out is that perhaps it could be another child whose organs are being donated to carry out these life-saving operations. It was always at the forefront of my mind, and it upset me greatly. But I knew that they more often than not used adult organs for children who needed a transplant simply because there were more available. That, to me, was less harrowing than if it was a child who had died.

So it was a week or so before we got home, having carried out all the different things they had to do before the transplant. Joanne had her 11th Birthday at home in September, and we managed to have a small celebration on the day. I had also been in touch with a charity called Dreams Come True who, among other things, arranged for sick children to meet their idols. I had written to them a few months prior to

Joanne's health deteriorating saying that Joanne was a big fan of Jason Donovan (and still was when she passed) and asked if there was any possibility of her getting to meet him. Shortly before her birthday I got a phone call out of the blue from the charity saying that Jason was coming to Glasgow to open a new venue – The Royal Concert Hall – later in the month. They asked if it was possible for Joanne to come along that night to see the show and meet with Jason after. I didn't hesitate in saying yes, so was told I would get a phone call nearer the date (25th September) to finalise arrangements. I kept it a secret from Joanne, and had planned to make sure she had plenty of rest near to the date so that she would be fit enough to enjoy the show.

The weekend before the show, we enjoyed a warm sunny day in the garden. When we were indoors later, the phone rang. As it was getting nearer the time of Jason's visit to Glasgow, I assumed that the lady with the English accent on the other end of the phone was calling from the charity with the last minute details of our trip to the concert on the following Tuesday. So I was shocked to hear it was a transplant co-ordinator phoning from Addenbrookes Hospital in Cambridge to tell us they had an organ for Joanne. I almost dropped the phone. I was in a complete panic. We were to wait for a taxi to come and pick us up to take us to Glasgow airport, where an air ambulance would be waiting for us. We did not need to arrange anything. Just get some things together for our stay in Cambridge. Oh God, Oh God, Oh God. Joanne was sitting in front of the TV with her friend Mhairi from next door. John was in the shower after doing a bit of gardening. I was panicking! Right. Calm down. Breathe. Think. Ok, this is it. I actually managed to calm down. I sat and waited for John to come out of the shower. I went upstairs and although I had a small case always at the ready with toiletries and things in case of a dash to the hospital, I asked John to get down the larger cases as we would all need to pack! Why had I not thought to pack before now! I didn't think it would be so soon, that's why. It was only three weeks since we had left the hospital in Cambridge.

I went back downstairs, bracing myself to speak to Joanne about the phone call and her first response was that she didn't want to go. Ok, fair enough. Neither did I! But that wasn't an option. So between us, John and I managed to turn it around, telling her how well she would be after the op. and all the exciting things we would do when she was feeling better. So for the next hour or so she busied herself packing her case full of stuff that, as it turned out, she would never use. Shellsuits were all the rage at the time, and she had one in every colour as well as matching boots. They all went in her case. As well as about 20 barbie dolls and umpteen other toys she wouldn't even look at. She put in loads of video tapes which it turned out did get used. After her operation(s), when she was finally on the mend, it became a thing that the night staff would end up in Joanne's room watching Scotch n Wry, Francie and Josie, and Rab C Nesbitt. Word got round the hospital, and we found we had different staff visiting during their break just to see the video tapes. It became a big thing – they all thought our Scottish humour was hilarious.

Around 9 o'clock that night, the taxi arrived to take us to the airport. Our family and neighbours had gathered in our front room, all trying to make sure that Joanne was not too traumatised before leaving.

We arrived at Glasgow airport a short time later. Away from the main entrance to the airport we were taken to where the air ambulances were kept in hangars. As we passed each one, they seemed to get smaller and smaller! We were met by a nurse and the pilot. The plane was tiny – only room for a stretcher type bed and three seats around the bed, with the pilot up front on his own. Oddly, I thought, there were five aeroplane meals stacked in a corner on board as well. But when the nurse offered us food during our flight, the only person to accept was Joanne. I recall she polished off three of the meals, saying "well I won't get anything to eat for a while".

For the first time in my life I can honestly say that I had no fear of flying. I was too worried about what lay ahead! As we approached the runway on our descent into Stansted airport, I could see the flashing lights of an ambulance and police car on the tarmac awaiting our arrival. We arrived at Addenbrookes' Hospital in the early hours after another blue light ambulance journey and a police escort. When we got her settled onto the ward, Joanne was examined and prepared for her transplant later that morning.

Anyone who has a child in need of an operation can identify with me on this, but handing over your child to a stranger to perform surgery on your child – albeit in an attempt to fix them - is the worst feeling in the world. No matter how necessary it is, it is your worst nightmare. And the guilt you feel is just horrendous. But I can honestly say that Joanne went without a word and without a tear. She was the bravest, most courageous person I have ever met. Why couldn't it be me on that bed instead of her?

They told us that transplants normally took around 6 hours. So we waited, going for walks around the hospital, sitting in the café, then the restaurant, then back to the ward for any news, and then doing it all again. The hospital at Addenbrookes has the biggest concourse I have seen in any hospital I have visited. It is almost the size of a shopping mall, with a good few shops and places to eat. There is a bank, clothes shop, newsagents, flower shop, travel shop, hairdressers, McDonalds, KFC, tea shop, restaurant, café among many others. But your mind is on the operation, so you find yourself just wandering aimlessly for most of the time, and nothing can take your mind off what is happening to your child. You can't eat, and most of the time you just feel sick with worry. When the six hours were up, we couldn't wait to get back to the ward to ask if they could check with theatre about how things were going. The news wasn't great. They had just got the old liver out, and it would be a while yet before Joanne would be out of surgery. It turned out to be another six hours before Joanne's operation was finally over, and another hour before she was taken from theatre to the intensive care unit.

The relief of just knowing that she had come through the operation was enormous, but we had to wait a while in a side room to speak to the surgeon. When he arrived, Peter Johnstone looked totally exhausted. At the forefront of my mind, I had to ask if the donor organ came from another child. It was my first question. When he told me it had, I just burst into tears. I was so distraught that a child had died that day, and had given my child the chance of life. All the while when Joanne was in theatre, I had this overwhelming feeling of hopelessness – I couldn't do anything to change this situation or make it better, it was all beyond my control. And I thought so much about the family who had just lost a loved one, and who, despite this, had thought about organ donation. I thought about their loss, not knowing whether or not we were going to lose Joanne, and the thought that it might be another child bothered me so much. Although Joanne had come through the operation, it was just the start of a long and difficult recovery for her. So although relieved that she had come this far, I still feared what the future might hold.

Mr Johnstone was a youngish father of two small children himself, so he knew exactly where I was coming from. He was a well-known kidney transplant surgeon in New Zealand, and had come over to England to learn about liver transplants, and after a couple of years living and working in Cambridge he had become one of their best surgeons in this field. He explained how the procedure was not straightforward in Joanne's case, because of her complications, and that he had to do the operations "a bit differently". So, of course, in our eyes he was the best, because he had successfully carried out what we knew would be a very difficult job! But in those days there was still Professor Cahn working away in the hospital – he was the surgeon who pioneered liver transplantation in Britain – and so he was still considered number one.

Seeing your child in intensive care after a liver transplant is quite a traumatic experience. So much so, that the hospital had published a booklet with graphic photographs of all the equipment necessary to keep your child alive in the first two or three days after their transplant. Usually patients are attending clinics for a while before they have their operation, and they are given all this information, but Joanne's had happened so quickly that we didn't get any of the information and so we weren't prepared for what was to come. When we were led into the intensive care unit that night, Joanne was in a "bubble" room, where no one was allowed to enter unless completely gowned up and scrubbed clean within an inch of their lives. It was rather futuristic in those days. But it was still the very early stages of liver transplants in children, so they were super careful when it came to post- operative aftercare.

Gradually, some of the equipment began to disappear, and we were allowed in beyond the glass barrier that separated us from Joanne. Immediately, I noticed that her eyes were white and not green! I had never in the whole of her life seen her eyes look so bright. And they looked huge. She looked beautiful!

To us, Joanne seemed to be making good progress, so after a few of days John dropped the bombshell that he would have to go home to check up on things at home and with work, and thought it would be a good idea to do so when my two brothers and my mum were coming down to visit that weekend. I wasn't happy about this, as we still did not know if Joanne was out of the woods so to speak. But he was insistent, and I couldn't be bothered arguing. I should have known then that he wasn't coping and needed to escape. But he had always been very good at hiding his fears and not talking about them – always putting on a front – always saying everything would be ok to me and Joanne. And to be honest, we believed it because he said it with such conviction and was so sure that he made us believe it. Really, though, deep down he was as scared as we were.

So while my two brothers and my mum were travelling down to visit us in hospital, John made his way back home. While doing his ward round one day, Mr Johnstone had mentioned that he wasn't entirely happy with Joanne's progress, but thought it might just be because she had been so ill before the operation and she was taking a bit longer to progress. I phoned John with the news, and told him to get right back to the hospital. I knew this wasn't going well. My gut feeling since the operation was that it wasn't done and dusted.

I asked my brothers to take my mum back home when they were leaving although the intention had been that she would wait with me until John arrived back. She was struggling to cope. She hadn't expected it to be quite so harrowing, and it was stressing me more that she was so upset by it all.

So I was on my own with Joanne until John arrived back the following Friday night. On the Saturday morning we had just left Joanne's bedside to go for a coffee, when two doctors sitting near us in the café immediately jumped up and ran off after being paged. I overheard one say to a passing doctor "Joanne's going back into theatre" and they all headed off, running towards the lift to get to the operating suite. You can imagine the size of this hospital when I say there were over 6000 staff members. But we just knew that out of all the patients there, these doctors were talking about our Joanne. We ran back to the intensive care, to be told that Mr Johnstone had decided on his ward round that he decided to do an exploratory operation.

The hospital was a teaching hospital, so there were lots of people watching the operation from beyond a glass partition, just as there had been at her transplant. As it turned out, Mr Johnstone was right to be concerned as Joanne's body was rejecting the liver, and he had to cut away the part of the new liver which was dying off inside her body in order to save her life. Another four hours of surgery.

Joanne's deterioration continued after this operation, and she had to be taken back to theatre the following Tuesday evening for the same procedure – cutting away another part of the liver. We waited outside the theatre, and followed the dozen or so staff who were holding up all sorts of drips and machinery while she was transported back to the intensive care unit after her op. With all these doctors and nurses surrounding her and transferring all her equipment over from the portable ones, Joanne's heart stopped. Immediately the ward sister jumped onto the bed and started pounding her heart. We were pushed outside the room while they tried frantically to save Joanne's life. It was some time later we were allowed to go back in to her bedside. She had been stabilised, but for the first time ever, the Sister came to our side and offered us a "drink for your nerves – what would you like?"

We knew things were bad when we were being offered alcohol, but Steve had always said "don't panic unless you see me panicking", and to be honest we hadn't noticed that as yet. And we weren't aware of the full extent of her condition. Joanne had developed sepsis after her transplant.

On the Thursday morning as we sat at Joanne's bedside in intensive care, Steve breezed through the door and pointing at Joanne "I've got you a new liver" was all he said as he passed the bottom of her bed. But almost immediately after the words left his mouth, all I could hear was the sound of the nurses sobbing! They all came round the bed in floods of tears, hugging John and I. I honestly hadn't noticed there was so much tension around us, but Steve's next words to me were "did you not see me panicking?"

So later in the afternoon, I was giving Joanne a bed bath to prepare her for surgery. From the corner of the room the Sister asked if anyone would like tea and a piece of carrot cake. Joanne was lying there with her oxygen mask on, unable to speak, but with a cheeky grin her hand shot up in the air. It certainly broke the tension for a bit, the staff couldn't believe she still had her sense of humour.

For the fourth time in less than three weeks, Joanne was once again taken into theatre, this time for her second transplant. We decided to go into town for a change of scene and to pass the first couple of hours or so. We didn't feel any less worried about things, you never get used to it no matter how many times you have been there and you never get complacent about the outcome.

This transplant took over 6 hours. It wasn't so difficult to remove the old liver this time round as it hadn't really settled in place. And so here we were, back in the intensive care, waiting and hoping and praying that this time it would be okay.

And so it was. This was an adult's liver this time, and somehow I didn't feel so bad about that. Obviously we had a lot to thank the donor's family for, and would be eternally grateful for what they had done, but all I mean is that as it wasn't another child it seemed to make it a bit more bearable. Even before Joanne's first transplant, I always wished there was an alternative to this – a man-made organ perhaps. It is a tragedy that this is the only option, but people need to be assured that organ recipients are not waiting for someone to die so that they can live, believe me. They don't wish to be sick in the first place, and if there was another option I am sure they would take it first.

A slow recovery, but Joanne went from strength to strength with no major hiccups. It was November now, and she had spent most of the last 5 months in hospital. She had to have a lot of physio, and practically had to learn to walk again, but she was getting there. The transplant team had done an amazing job, but even so when it was time to go home, we almost ran out the door. There was medication that Joanne would have to take for the rest of her life, and there would be plenty of visits back to Cambridge, but my God, was it worth it all. To see this little girl, sitting in the taxi on our way to the train station – her eyes were as bright as her teeth! And they looked HUGE. No yellow skin and no green eyes – for the first time in her life! She was just beautiful. And healthy. And perfect.

9

We came home to a tremendous welcome. Honestly, friends and family just wouldn't stay away. Our house was full every day. We had visitors all the time – everyone just wanted to keep checking to make sure she was still ok. It really was hard to believe the transformation. She had to use a wheelchair outdoors for a couple of months, but after that there was no stopping her. She soon went back to school, and loved being the centre of attention for a while. But really all she ever wanted to do was to be "normal".

So with her new-found strength and improved health, one of her ambitions was to learn to swim. She hadn't ever been scared of the water, (as I am) and enjoyed splashing around when we were on holidays, but she wanted to go to the local swimming pool and learn to swim properly. Sandra and Pamela Ross were the two daughters of our friends and neighbours, Ian and Eileen Ross. The girls were like big sisters to Joanne, and so they volunteered to take her to the baths and teach her to swim. It wasn't something John and I could get involved in as John wasn't much of a swimmer and I had a fear in the water and couldn't swim at all. But Joanne wasn't long in getting to grips with it, and soon we were to find that it would come in handy!

On one of our visits to Addenbrookes ' for a check-up we were told that the Transplant Games were to be held in Glasgow in the summer time, and Joanne was asked if she would like to take part and be in the Cambridge team. She thought about swimming right away, and said yes.

So less than one year after her transplants, Joanne took part in the swimming events at the Maryhill Swimming Pool, and ended up with a silver medal. All the events at the Games were being covered by the Press, and it was challenged by one of the photographers from Glasgow when Joanne was announced as "Joanne Brannigan from Cambridge". He had recognised her from a previous article he did the photos for in the Sunday Mail, and declared in front of everyone, "naw she's no – she's fae Glesca". He was also the first to challenge the result when Joanne got her silver medal, claiming that the winner was "cheating". Think she had a fan there.

Later that year, on Joanne's 12th Birthday, I came home from work early as we had arranged to go out for a celebratory meal. I was met by Joanne who came running down the path screaming "I'm going to America". "Really" I replied "Who with?" (knowing full well that I could never go on a plane for longer than 3 hours). "Honestly mum, I'm going to America" she said, dragging me by the hand into the house. John was standing in the front room reading a letter. "show mum" she told him. "I've just opened it, but it's a letter from "Dreamflight" he said. "Joanne has been nominated by Addenbrookes to go to Disneyworld in America in November. I'm just reading it again to make sure that I read it correctly ". Dreamflight is a charity organised by staff of British Airways. They do fundraising all year round so that they can take a planeload of sick children for a visit to Disneyworld. Most of the children are either terminally ill or chronically sick, and there are plenty of escorts, including doctors and nurses, who volunteer to go along with the British Airways staff to look after them. The holiday was to take place in November and would be for 10 days. Joanne was again part of the Cambridge team, and was paired up with a girl she had met in Addenbrookes, Anna Rawling from Cornwall. We had met Anna and her family at the hospital, and we all seemed to hit it off. The staff in the hospital who nominated the girls knew that they had become friends, and so thought it would work for them to be together while they were away.

Joanne flew down to London from Glasgow to be met and escorted to the hotel by one of the BA staff. There she met up with Anna. Before she left us at Glasgow Airport, it was all a bit tearful, and she was having a change of heart about going, but she agreed to wait til she met up with Anna and see how she felt then. There was a party arranged for all the children that night in the hotel they were staying in overnight before their departure to America the next day, and there were lots of special guests like Ant and Dec (although they were PJ and Duncan then) who would be there to meet the children and join in the party.

The following morning Joanne phoned from the hotel, full of excitement. She had loved the party, and was getting on great with

Anna. They had met with their escort, a handsome young doctor they were to call "Higgy" – Dr Higginson. So that was that. All the uncertainty and us parents forgotten already! Did she not realise we had never been apart before? Did she not know that this was traumatising for us parents? Clearly not!

I think I sank into a state of depression while she was away – honestly. The house was so quiet without her. I hadn't actually realised she was so noisy. So chatty. So full of life. Not until she wasn't there. The house was dead without her. Just as well we had work to go to, kept our minds occupied and passed the time til she got back.

So on the day of her arrival home, John went to pick her up at the airport while I was at work. When she came running in to greet me at the office, she looked totally shattered. But she loved every minute of it. She had so many souvenirs, and Higgy made sure that there were plenty of photographs on her camera. So the whole Dreamflight trip was the topic of conversation for the next few weeks. Honestly, she just totally loved it. Who would have thought she would ever be capable of doing such a thing just over a year ago. It was beyond our wildest dreams. But once she had a taste of this, there was no stopping her.

A couple of weeks after her return, the Dreamflight team sent us more souvenirs of their holiday, including a photograph album and video. Everyone said she was a star, happy and smiley all the time, except when it was time to say goodbye to everyone. The video showed just how much all the children had enjoyed the holiday, but it was Joanne who was in tears when she had to leave them all, and so that was what they decided to show at the very end of the video – Joanne's teary face. Anna became a lifelong friend, visiting here in Scotland for short holidays and Joanne visiting Anna and her family in Cornwall and later in London when Anna went to university there. They had a strong bond, Anna and Joanne, and found it easy to relate to one another. They also met up from time to time in Cambridge as the doctors would often try to make their appointments for the same day. They would go to the same clinic there for a few years after their transplants and were always made warmly welcome by the doctors and nurses. On one visit, Joanne was met by Steve who by this time was married and had moved from London to live in Cambridge. "I'm just popping home to feed the dog" he said "want to come?". And so Joanne duly wandered off with her consultant to go to his house to feed his dog instead of sitting in the waiting room with us to attend her transplant clinic appointment!

So now from the age of 12 Joanne had decided that this new life of hers was not going to be wasted. Don't get me wrong, it wasn't a bad life she had before, and she always said that she didn't know how sick she was as a child, she just thought it was normal to feel tired and lethargic most of the time. But after her transplants she had so much more energy, and she wasn't going to let it go to waste. Early the following year I received a call from the Dreams Come True charity asking how Joanne was and also if she would be well enough to come down to London to meet Jason since she had missed out when he was in Glasgow. He was appearing in the west end show Joseph and His Amazing Technicolour Dreamcoat at the London Palladium. Naturally I said I would get her there no matter what. And so shortly after I had to tell her in advance that we were going to London to meet Jason. She was ecstatic, and couldn't wait to plan the trip. She wanted her hair permed – it was the fashion then! – and needed a new wardrobe of course. So shopping it was then. Unfortunately, the perm came out rather curlier than she wanted – think the medication she was on might have had something to do with it. But it didn't stop her – she was going to meet Jason by hook or by crook although she still blamed me for many years to come for letting her get that damned perm! We were put up in a nice hotel at Piccadilly in London during our stay, and on the first night made our way to the theatre. We were met by a representative from the charity, along with a few other sick children and their families. We had front row seats, where Joanne sat in awe of her idol's performance during the show. After the show, Jason came out to the front to meet with the children and chat to each individually. Unfortunately Joanne was completely dumb struck and could hardly say her name. But give him his due, he did try to have a conversation with her, and complemented her no end on her fashion sense and hairstyle. Then we had some photographs taken with him. Truly a memorable evening, and Joanne never stopped being a huge Jason fan after that.

Her teenage years were, for the most part, fairly normal. She was just as stroppy at times, as most teenagers are. John always said it was only her and I that clashed though. At one point I thought to myself – don't like her but still love her! Thankfully this phase didn't last long, and she was soon back to being her lovely self.

It was when she was about 15 years old that my mum came to stay with us. She had been suffering from dementia for a few years, and was now becoming quite confused and agitated, so when a small flat was for sale near our home, we decided to buy it for mum to make life easier for us all. While we were getting the flat ready for her to move in, she stayed with us in our home. Having company of others around her seemed to help her a lot, she seemed less agitated. I transferred to another job within the council with reduced hours, so I went out to work only two and a half days a week. We soon got into a routine on the days I was at work -John was able to pop up to the house during the day to make sure mum was ok and make her a cuppa and something to eat. It wasn't something we had discussed, but Joanne took over her nightly routine of helping her with having a bath and getting her ready for bed. I could hear them chatting away and laughing when they spent this time together. There was no awkwardness on Joanne's part that their roles were reversed and she was now looking after her nana. I was then left to keep up with her washing, making sure she had a clean outfit on each day and doing her hair. Not as easy as it sounds, as mum would often put dirty clothes back in the drawer beside clean clothes so every night I would spend washing and ironing a drawer full of clothes. But our routines were working like magic, and I can honestly say that mum's last days spent living with us were the happiest she had been in a long time. And it showed me that my beautiful daughter was growing into a very caring as well as loving young lady.

She still wasn't that interested in academic work at school, but she was interested in looking after and caring for people. When it came to decide what she wanted to do as a career, she had thought about working with children in a nursery or older people in care. She tried the nursery first, but decided that it didn't really suit her – she found it a bit too noisy! While she was still at school and old enough to take a job, her dad managed to help get her work cleaning in the local high school after school hours. She was over the moon that she was earning money while still at school, and a couple of her friends soon followed her into doing the same job. It meant that they still had their weekends free, so it certainly suited them better than a Saturday job! Joanne was still doing this work while considering what she wanted to do as a "proper" job, and working for the local authority she had access to the "job bulletins" which were circulated round the various council establishments. When there was a job advertised internally to clean in a house for adults with learning difficulties, Joanne immediately applied to be transferred there. She was interviewed shortly after and her application was successful.

She was totally taken with the whole concept of adults who were maybe not able to look after a house or themselves being helped to do so while living with others in the same situation. It made sense. They had their own individual personalities, so sometimes it didn't go swimmingly, but hey that's the same in any "family". Part of the house was lived in by those who needed a lot of help on a daily basis, and another part was lived in by others who didn't need much help at all, but could come to the staff for assistance or just for a chat any time they needed to. It was a good mix of people. The property wasn't too large either – three terraced council houses that had been knocked together as one and adapted to suit the residents with easy access throughout, so it was a good set-up.

But it was the people that really pulled at Joanne's heartstrings. She just loved working there, and enjoyed chatting to them. It wasn't long before she would come home with stories of what they were getting up to – playing their favourite music and dancing and singing, playing games and just having fun. Most had a routine of going to the centre for adults with learning difficulties and other clubs too. There was also the serious side of trying to help them with chores associated with every day living, do meaningful activities, and developing as people, as well as providing emotional support when they were feeling out of sorts or a bit down. It wasn't an easy job – they all had different needs. But it made sense to Joanne that after a while of cleaning in the house, she decided that she wanted to be a Support Worker for Adults with Learning Difficulties. And so when a suitable job came up, she applied and was successful.

Her natural instincts and her times in and out of hospitals helped her to understand what was needed for this type of work. She realised the importance of building relationships with each individual, and establishing what support they each needed. She was so caring and loving, so her disposition made the job easy for her to adapt to. There were elements of the job she wasn't particularly fond of – like all the paperwork – but her natural instincts to care and help people who were less fortunate had drawn her to this type of work. Over the years, she cared for many individuals in different homes run by the council and worked with many different colleagues, some of whom became great friends. It is not encouraged to have a friendship or any sort of relationship with the people you are looking after in this type of job, the emphasis on remaining professional, but Joanne always felt that spending so much time with them in their home, she wanted to create a good friendly and caring atmosphere for them to thrive. So from what I know of her at her work, when appropriate, she was focused on developing a relationship with each person individually, interested in keeping it "fun", and was all for having a laugh and joke with them.

Not long after my mum passed away, I began to feel unwell. To be frank, I probably had felt a bit lethargic before mum died, but put it down to circumstances at that time. Anyway, I eventually went along to the doctor, and he was of the same mind – my symptoms were probably caused by grief and a lifetime of anxiety caused by Joanne's condition catching up with me. But he wanted to keep an eye on my progress, so I made regular appointments to see him at his surgery – either weekly or fortnightly.

I tried to carry on as best as I could, but when I was so sick one day that I couldn't take Joanne for a hospital appointment (she was around 15 years old and this was the first time in her life that I hadn't managed to go with her for a hospital appointment) I knew that there was something more serious going on. I had been keeping my regular appointments with my GP and keeping him up to date with any new symptoms, but I just wasn't getting any better – in fact I was getting worse. It wasn't that he was ignoring me because he did have a few tests carried out, but he just felt that I was emotionally spent and completely drained.

During this time, John telephoned my GP to speak to him, but as he was on holiday, he spoke to one of the other doctors in the practice.

I was by this time back working full time, and had started vomiting every morning before I left for work. I was also sleeping on the floor most nights when I got in from work, curled up in a ball on the rug in front of the fire for warmth, and John had to carry me upstairs to my bed because I was so exhausted. The doctor gave me a sick line for a month to see if a complete rest would help.

It was now almost a year after I had first went to see the original GP when during a visit he said he would like to do further blood tests. It was then I informed him that he had never actually taken any blood before then. I could see he was horrified at this, and watching him read back my notes I could see that he was becoming more concerned. He sent off the bloods, saying that some could take a wee while to come back. I told him we had a holiday booked and were leaving later that week. I could hear the panic in his voice when he said he would ask for them to be done urgently. The very next day he phoned me to tell me that I had no blood! He asked me to come to the surgery right away for injections and medication. This treatment was based on only some of the test results and he was hoping that he would have more results before we left for our holiday. He hadn't said I shouldn't go – but I hadn't asked! So by the end of the week, with no further contact from him, we left on our holidays.

The holiday went ok. It wasn't great – I suppose I had expected to have a new lease of life. But that didn't happen. I had a bit of trouble walking. My legs were like lead, and the iron tablets and sunshine weren't giving me renewed energy as I had hoped. On our return home two weeks later, there was a letter in the mail from the GP. Just a couple of lines, keeping it light. "Have made arrangements for you to see Dr. Carmichael, a consultant at the local hospital – don't panic!" Had heard these words before when Joanne was in Addenbrookes ' hospital, ,so it didn't bode well.

I telephoned the doctors' surgery and asked to speak to my GP. He was off on holiday, so I was put through to one of the other partners in the practice. Had he read the results of my recent blood tests and what did they indicate was wrong? He was a bit hesitant in giving me straightforward answers to my questions, so I just came out with it – could it indicate cancer? "Well, yes", he said "among other things it is a possibility".

John took me for my appointment, and when Dr. Carmichael, the consultant based at our local hospital, examined me, and immediately arranged for some x rays and scans to be done. There was a lengthy waiting list, he said, but why not pop round to the x ray department and see if they have any cancellations. We did, and as it happened, a woman I had been in school with called Marjory Walker was working there at the time. She was at the reception desk when we arrived, and after a quick catch-up, she said they would "squeeze me in tomorrow". Excellent. So the next day I was back at our local hospital having the scans and x rays carried out.

When John dropped me off later at the house, he went back to work and immediately telephoned Dr. Carmichael. Although he didn't have the results so quickly, he said he would phone round and get a verbal report on them. Shortly after he phoned John back and said there was something sinister showing, but I would need to go to another hospital to have a CAT scan, saying again there would probably be a bit of a wait before it could be done. John asked if he would phone the other hospital to see if there were any cancellations there, and he duly did. He was back within the hour saying I could have it done on the Friday provided we could arrange transport. Not a problem.

On the Friday after my scan, John phoned Dr. Carmichael again, asking him to phone the hospital for a verbal report on the scan. He duly did and came back with another appointment for me to go speak to him the following week.

When we went for this appointment, I was seen by another consultant, Mr Fletcher Dean, who had travelled down from Gartnaval Hospital in Glasgow especially to see me. "do you want the good news or the bad news first?" he asked. Give me the bad news first, I replied. Ok, so you have a tumour on your left kidney. It's rather large, and has probably been there for some time – years in fact. The good news is that your right kidney is working well, so we'll just take the left one out and see how things go from there. I wasn't expecting that – I honestly thought I was finished, and only went along with it all to see how much time I had left. So although the nurses thought I should be upset, I was actually quite the opposite. The operation was to be arranged within the next week or two, and he was apologetic that I would have to go to Glasgow to have it done. I would have gone anywhere to get this sorted to get back to normal!

As it turned out, I was gravely ill by the time I was taken in to hospital to have my operation. I had no blood and it was touch and go whether or not I would be well enough to withstand the operation. Despite having a blood transfusion over a couple of days shortly after my admission, the anaesthetist came round the night before my operation was scheduled for, and told me that I would not come through the operation alive. She suggested that she be given more time to get my blood up to levels that would give me a fighting chance. So I agreed to postpone the operation for another couple of days. Mr Dean was not happy when he heard, as he felt I was running out of time. So it really was a catch 22 situation. But two days after the operation was originally scheduled, I had my left kidney removed – along with a massive tumour – and survive I did.

Joanne was a star throughout all of this time. She couldn't do enough for me, and unknown to me at the time, she was also working behind the scenes trying to keep John's spirits up too. He had told her that I might not make it and she often found him in tears. I can't take anything away from John because he was amazing too, but most of the time I was oblivious to what was going on and was totally unaware that they were propping each other up.

It was after the operation that my mental health actually did suffer. Depression took over. I wasn't recovering quickly enough, and it was frustrating watching John and Joanne going out to work in the morning, and I could hardly lift a hoover! But there was this team effort thing going on. As well as doing a full time job, John was doing all the housework, laundry, shopping and looking after me. Joanne was his wingman.

But I had no strength. I was tired all the time, and sometimes I physically felt a whole lot worse than I had before the operation. My brain was working, and that was telling me I was useless! And I didn't have my mum. I don't think I got the chance to mourn her death, as I was ill at the time, without realising how ill I was. And now I missed her so much, but at the same time I was glad she hadn't lived to see me like this.

So it took a couple of years, a lot of frustration and a lot of ups and downs before I finally got my act together and got back on track. I found myself a part time job, and things gradually got back to normal. Thank God Joanne was in good health during this period of our lives.

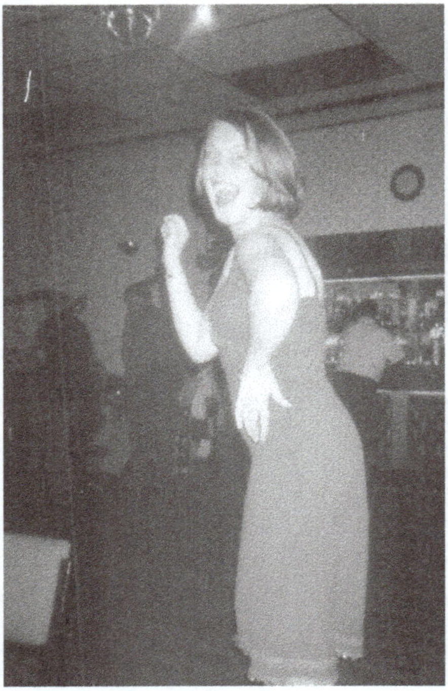

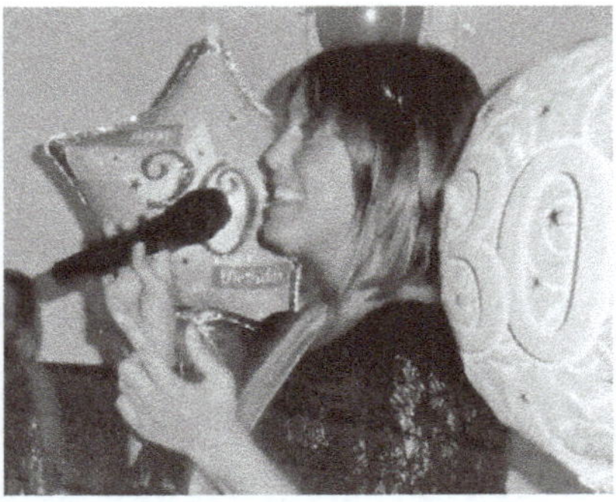

Can't believe I'm 30

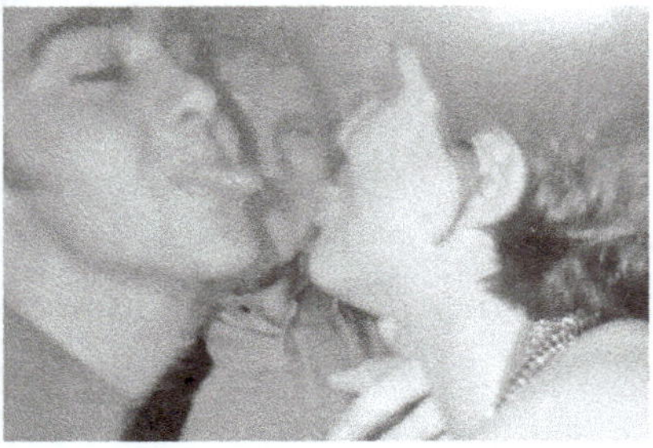

Happy Birthday to me!

Me and my mad mate Gary

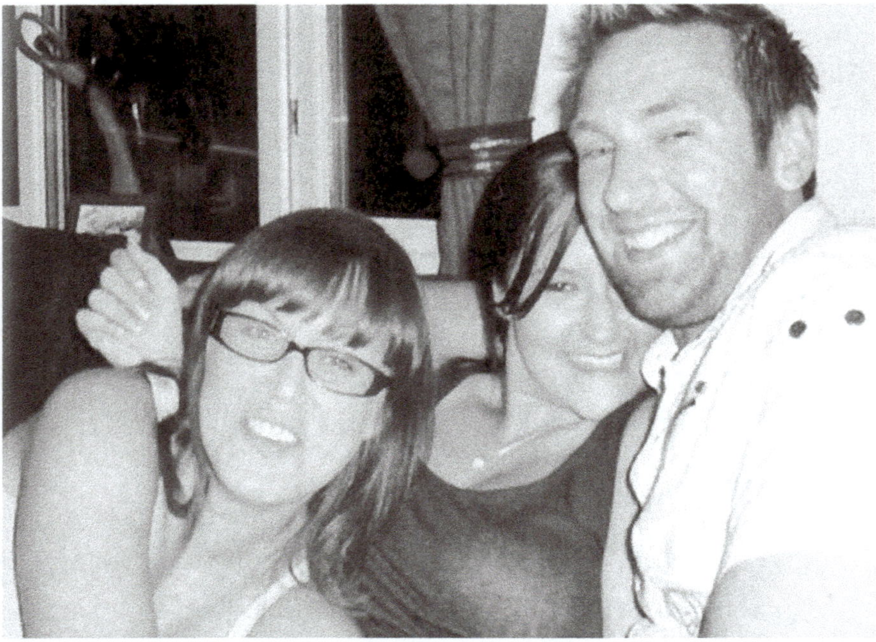

A wee night in with Nicola and David

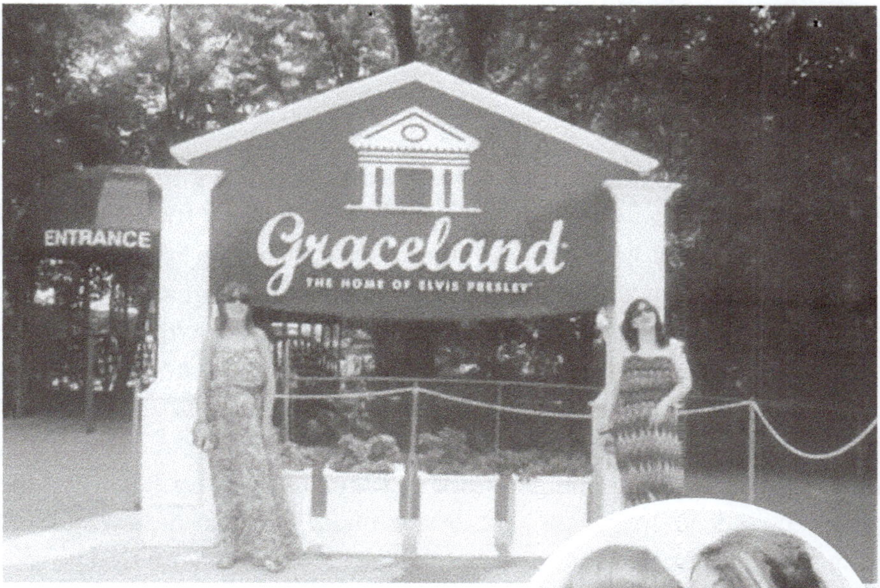

With Laura in Memphis, the home of the blues, rock 'n' roll and Beale Street. Woo Hoo!

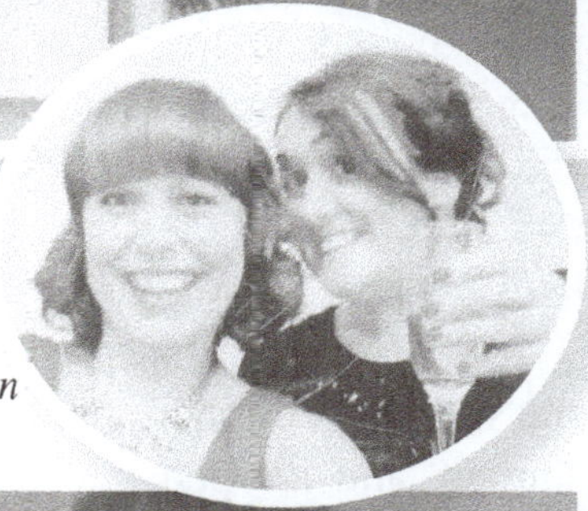

Celebrating with Alison

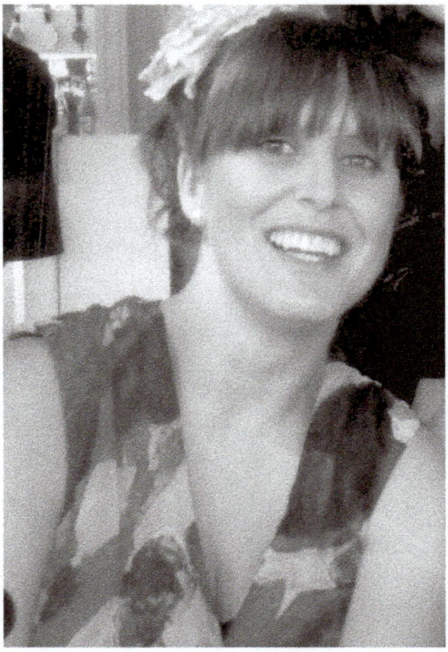

Celebrating Nicola and David's wedding

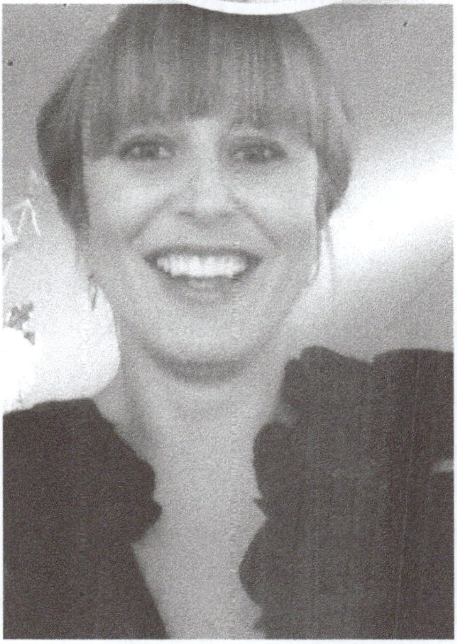

Celebrating Sharon and Mick's wedding

10

Just before her 17th birthday Joanne asked if she could go on her first holiday abroad with just her friends. There were four of them all together, and they were looking at a two week holiday on Majorca. I was thinking she was still too young, and was reluctant to say yes, but when one of the other mums said she would go along with a friend and stay at the same apartments, we all agreed to let them go.

To say they had a ball is an understatement. They met up with a group of lads from Huddersfield who lived in the same apartment building. A couple of the guys noticed that Joanne mostly lay at the pool covered up during the day. It was really hot, and they wondered why she wasn't going into the pool. When they asked her why, she said she had a huge scar on her body from her operations. Mr Johnstone had made a point of opening her scar up at the same point for each of her operations, so it wasn't as bad as it could have been.

The boys said that it was something she should be proud of, and she shouldn't think about what others thought. They lifted her off the sunbed, and jumped into the pool while holding onto Joanne. She wasn't annoyed – she was always up for a laugh and in fact it was just what she needed. They had told her that the scar was a symbol of what she had been through, and she should never hide it from anyone. Her badge of honour! From then on, she never covered up and if anyone stared it didn't bother her in the slightest.

The girls went back to the same apartments the following year, arranging to meet up with the boys again. This was followed by a visit down to Huddersfield. Although they never met up again after that Joanne kept in touch with a couple of them from time to time over the next 20 years, Dave Barclay and Naeem Mohammed, and this became more regular through Facebook.

There were other holidays with her friends that followed, one year after the other. She became a bit of a social animal, enjoying nights out, parties and gigs.

She was hanging out with a group of friends who were only interested in their cars, and that proved to be a good thing because they weren't bothered about drinking. They would meet up in a local bar most nights, but just to play pool, and usually went to the cinema or gigs in Glasgow each week too. Joanne started taking driving lessons herself around this time, but clearly she had too many "chauffeurs" for her to stick at it. It wasn't until it was coming up to her 21st birthday that we thought we would buy her a wee runaround car, just to see if that would encourage her more to get back behind the wheel. Initially it did. She would often sit in it outside the house, music blaring, but wasn't in any hurry to start up her lessons again. As time went by though, she made up her own mind that she wanted to drive the damned thing, so she started taking lessons again. When we asked how she got on each time she came in from a lesson she usually had some juicy bit of gossip the instructor had given her, or a baking recipe, or where to go to get her hair or nails done! Eh. But what about the driving? Ok was the only response on that subject. Eventually she was told to put in for her driving test which she duly did. Five different driving instructors and six driving tests later, and a couple of years later, she PASSED. You see, she just couldn't master reversing round a corner, and of course she was given this to do in each of her driving tests. The last instructor told Joanne from day one that she could drive perfectly well, so he concentrated solely on her reversing round corners. He told her to forget how she had been taught in the past, and taught her a way that he felt was much easier to understand. And it worked. Joanne was never ashamed that it had taken her so many attempts to pass her test. She was in good company. "Hubby in her heid" – Ralf Little – took the same amount of driving tests before he passed.

After her operations in Cambridge and London, Joanne had to visit the hospitals there regularly for check-ups. Although John would come with us to Cambridge, it was mostly just Joanne and I who went to the hospital in London, as these visits soon included theatre breaks and shopping trips. It was, of course, Joanne who would check out what was on and what we would be doing while we were down there. London is an amazing city, and we always found the people there very helpful and kind. We made a point of not going to the same places on our visits but it isn't difficult to vary what you do and see when you are there. So it became a firm favourite of ours despite having to include the hospital appointments on our visits. I felt that, even when Joanne was very young, that it was important not to see going to hospital as a frightening thing, so I always planned a treat of some sort for us to do after each appointment, whether it was an important thing she was going for or just something minor we always followed it by going for lunch or a bit of retail therapy. As she got older it was Joanne who arranged what we would do after!

When she reached her teenage years, the doctors in Cambridge decided to transfer her case notes to the Royal Infirmary in Edinburgh, where they had by then opened a Liver Transplant unit for adults. Joanne hadn't been seen by the paediatric doctors in Cambridge for a couple of years now anyway, and so it made sense to visit the nearest hospital that could deal with her complex condition. Initially she alternated six monthly visits between Cambridge and Edinburgh and she no longer had to go to the hospital in London. Over time, her liver results were becoming less stable, and at the back of everyone's mind I suppose that we all felt that she would need further surgery. The problem with Joanne was that the medical professionals were not really sure what that might entail because of the complexities within her body.

But she carried on, dealing with the blows of life that assaulted her in her own individual way. Living her life as normally and as best she could. When it came to her 21st Birthday, we had arranged a surprise party at the local bowling green hall. Joanne was to arrive with her friends, on the pretence that they were going to someone else's party. I remember when we were told they would be arriving soon, so everyone was prepared for her entrance. At some point someone left the hall, leaving the door slightly ajar when she arrived with her friends. She later said she could see our neighbours Mary and Hughie sitting inside the hall, and wondered how on earth they knew this other person who was supposedly holding the party. But within seconds, she was in the room and initially in complete shock when everyone cheered and began singing "Happy Birthday". I could see the tears forming in her eyes. She was overcome. After hugging and kissing her dad and I, she left us standing as she made her way round the whole hall, thanking everyone for coming. That's just how she was. Always grateful and gracious. You can't teach that. It was in her soul.

11

It wasn't long after her 21st Birthday that we had our next big medical problem to face though. It was John's turn! On Christmas day he complained of feeling unwell, and decided to have an early night. He had been complaining of indigestion on and off throughout the day but it hadn't stopped him eating a huge Christmas Dinner and other goodies beside. He got up during the night – still complaining of indigestion – but duly went downstairs and had more cheese and crackers.

Early next morning, in the light of day, I did notice that he looked rather grey, so we agreed he should go to the hospital to get checked out. Sure enough, he was having a heart attack. Luckily it was mild, and so he was kept in hospital over the next few days to recover. The doctors decided that he would have to have an angioplasty at a later date. Time passed, and it was more than ten months later before he actually had the operation. The delay, they said, was due to an oversight. Although the operation is fairly straightforward, John became unwell shortly after his discharge from the hospital in Glasgow where he had had the procedure. He was still recovering at home from the op. so I asked our GP to carry out a home visit. It was a locum who came out, and she advised us that John had a "viral infection" and prescribed an antibiotic. After a few days he seemed no better, so I called out the doctor again. Blood samples were taken, and we were to await the results. It was Christmas time again, and John was spending most of the time unwell in bed at home. It was a busy time for Joanne at work, and on Christmas day I found myself on my own because Joanne had to work and John was still bedridden. Christmas time is so emotional anyway, so I found myself sitting on my own crying my eyes out because I was so worried about everything – John was so ill and Joanne's health wasn't great either.

I calmed myself down, reminding myself how lucky we were. We had our troubles, but we got always managed to get through them. And so the day passed.

But the next day when I took some drinks and food up to John I couldn't get him to waken. When he did eventually open his eyes, he was not focusing well and as he spoke he wasn't making sense. He was always a bit of a joker, but I knew instinctively that he wasn't messing around. He was hallucinating, so I immediately telephoned the doctor and he organised an ambulance to take him to hospital, without even coming out to see him. At that time, we still had a local hospital with a consultant present at all times, so John was admitted into the High Dependency Unit there. Meanwhile some of the results of the blood samples which were taken a few days earlier were coming back through the system, and it was established that John had caught clostridium difficile – c.diff – in the hospital in Glasgow while he was there having the angioplasty. It was common knowledge to the hospital staff that it was going round the patients there at the time, but it wasn't really heard outwith the hospital community. His condition had worsened because the locum doctor had prescribed antibiotics before knowing what the infection was. So he spent the next six weeks in the local hospital where they tried desperately to make him well. Unfortunately they were not able to clear the infection and had to perform a colostomy operation to remove his bowel.

After the operation, he seemed to be progressing well, and it wasn't long before he was back home. He had lost so much weight and become so weak over the time he had spent in the hospital and so he had to use a wheelchair outside for a short while.

Although he had been through such a difficult time, John was never open about his true feelings and would never show or talk about how he really felt about it all. He liked to give the impression that he was just getting on with things, but really he wasn't coping at all. We had, after all, had many years of constant and serious health problems among each of us in the family, and John being the man of the house always felt that it was his role to carry the burden.

We went away for a few days just to take a break from things, and shortly after when he was strong enough, we had a holiday abroad. Joanne came along – she said in case I needed help, but I'm sure she just wanted to be there to see that her dad was ok. Joanne idolised her dad, and in her eyes he could do no wrong. But after that holiday even she could see that he was changing. He had never routinely gone to the pub for a pint, in fact he rarely did, preferring to have wine with a meal at weekends. But he began secretly drinking at home, and it wasn't long before his drinking habits became a problem for us all as a family. Along with this he became very depressed and isolated himself from the outside world and family life. His character completely changed and he lost interest in other things that were at one time important to him.

Joanne had moved into her own flat, not because of her dad but just because she wanted to have her own place to invite friends. It was nearby, so she still came home for her meals, depending on her shifts at work. She got herself a wee kitten for company. She was loving her independence and living her life to the full.

Over the next few years though, John's drinking was a difficult problem to deal with and I suppose it could have been handled differently if we had not been faced with the ongoing health problems Joanne had to face. Her liver results were becoming concerning, and she was spending more and more time in hospital. But it still wasn't stopping her carrying on with as normal a life as possible.

On one occasion when her blood count was low, our GP telephoned the consultant Dr Camichael at the local hospital to ask if she could pop in for a transfusion because she had a hen weekend to go to in Majorca! The nurse on the ward thought we were winding her up when we turned up the next day, but when she checked it out, sure enough there was a bed with Joanne's name on it.

She was getting on with her life – despite knowing she was becoming more and more sick again.

When she was about 25 years old, we went to Cambridge for checks, and she was kept in for a month. Not long after we got home, she took a sudden turn for the worse and became really unwell. She was transferred through to Edinburgh where they made the decision to put her back on the transplant list.

12

It was much more difficult for me this time around. John and I had split up, although we were still living under the same roof for a while. I had reached the end – there was no talking to him – John was drinking very heavily and he had given up on trying to stop. Early on in his downward spiral, he would often break down. After a heavy drinking binge, he promised so many times that it would not happen again. But of course it did. I have no doubt that he became this alien because he had become depressed due to the endless battles we had experienced in our household with ill health. Before, he was the cheery positive one. I was the worrier. Now, I had to put my fears to one side and put on my brave armour to see my daughter through this – something I had always feared and hoped we would never have to go through again. I had to be strong. In the past, there were times when I was able to take time to myself if things got too much. I couldn't do that this time around.

So I decided it was time to move on. Joanne had moved back into her room at the house, although she still had her flat to go back to when she was better. But it wasn't suitable for her right then as it was on the first floor of the building, and she found the stairs problematic. There was a complete communication breakdown with John and myself, and surprisingly he stopped talking to Joanne too.

So I found a house for Joanne and I to share while she waited for her operation. She needed a stable home. She needed peace and quiet, where she could rest without worrying about how her dad was. She always worried more about him than she did about herself. She was all too aware of the change in him, and despite her serious health condition, it didn't stop her from trying to help him. But he just wanted to bury his head in the sand and carry on with this new way of dealing with things.

So I was the only parent able to go through this with Joanne and I couldn't shield her this time round – she was an adult, so there was no hiding anything from her. That was the worst thing for me. I couldn't shield her. I couldn't tell her not to worry - that everything would be ok - because the doctors were always open and honest. It was more difficult too because she had to wait 18 months on the waiting list this time round, all the while her condition was deteriorating and she had become very ill. But the doctors wanted to wait to get her an almost perfectly compatible liver so that she would have a better chance of surviving longer after the procedure. She was no longer able to go to work, but the Council where she worked as a support worker were more than happy to keep her job open for her until she was fit to return to work.

Again we were back to doing things on her good days, and riding out the storms of the bad times. It wasn't easy, and it isn't easy for anyone waiting for a transplant. There is no certainty that you will get the operation, and if you are accepted onto the waiting list, you don't know when it will take place, nor if it will be successful. It is a very stressful time.

Joanne became very weak, and a couple of weeks before her third transplant at the age of 27 we contacted the local newspaper, highlighting the plight of people like her who were desperately waiting for an organ, and raising awareness of the lack of donor organs. Joanne knew how ill she was, and very bravely spoke up for other people who could benefit, believing that it was too late for her. Thousands of people in the UK are waiting for an organ at any given time. Some are so sick that they die before a suitable one can be found because there is still an acute shortage of donors on the Organ Donation Register. Choosing to donate organs is a very generous thing to do, and a lifeline to hundreds of sick people who depend on receiving one in order to live. People, quite naturally, worry that if their name is on the organ donor register then maybe when they are sick and in hospital that doctors will not try to save them. But that's simply not true. Doctors have a duty of care to save your life first and it will always be their priority to try to do that.

But if, despite their best efforts, death is inevitable, then donation may be discussed with the family and next of kin. From the family's point this must be the most horrendous thing to think about – especially if you do not know the wishes of the person who is dying or if it is your child. And there are many myths surrounding organ donation, e.g. if you are in a coma they could take your organs. But this is not true. The majority of deceased organ donors are patients who have been declared brain dead. That is not the same this as being in a coma. People can recover from a coma, but not from brain death. Another myth is when people think they may be too old. Well the oldest donor that I have heard of was 93! What matters is the health and condition of your organs when you die not the age. And organ recipients are not waiting for someone to die so that they can be saved. Trust me. The last thing that any sick person wants is to hear of another patient lose their life. But when it's time for the operation, they have to focus on what lies ahead, and not what has happened in the past to get to this stage. Believe me when I say this, Joanne never forgot what another family went through for her to live. There was no-one more grateful than her to have been given the chance to live a healthy life. And you know what, I think that made her all the more determined not to waste the lifeline she had been given.

Joanne lived with her liver problem and was aware of it from an early age. She accepted that she had to go to hospitals on a regular basis. However, it wasn't until she became an adult that she became aware that liver organ transplants carry a stigma that no other organ transplantation does. Some people jump to the conclusion that if an adult needs a new liver then they must have been either drinking heavily or have been misusing drugs, and in fact, a GP on meeting Joanne for the first time after her third liver transplant actually asked her whether it was alcohol or drugs that led to her needing a new liver! Clearly that particular doctor had not bothered to read her file!

Joanne read many articles and stories of people in need of transplants. Most were due to having contracted some illness or other during their lives or were born with a life-threatening condition like Joanne herself. But some were because what started as social drinking had spiralled out of control and turned into deep addiction, and I think she came to realise that some of these people weren't always in control of their fate. Possibly because of what she saw at home, and how alcohol had changed her dad. She had recognised that addiction was a very difficult thing to overcome. You can start with the world at your feet, and in the blink of an eye, your life will consist of depression, isolation, hospitalisation, despair and even suicide attempts. Ultimately, you have lost everything you ever held dear.

Some people can overcome their addiction before it has destroyed their body too. But sometimes it can leave damage beyond repair. And in these cases, when a transplant becomes necessary, then there has to be a period when the patient has shown that they are in recovery and are willing to work hard to improve their health in preparation for a transplant. Only then, will they be considered for inclusion on the transplant waiting list. It is a difficult decision for anyone to have to make. Who should have a second or third chance at life? Must it depend on how they have lived their lives? When the NHS seems to be in such financial difficulties and seriously under threat of being rationalised by political parties in Scotland and the rest of the UK, then how do medical professionals decide how funds should be spent? I certainly wouldn't like to make such decisions.

It worried Joanne so much when well known celebrities were in the news because their alcohol addiction had led to their having a liver transplant. It was often the case that they were not a good advert for transplantation, especially when the gift of an organ did not stop them carrying on with their lifestyle. Some people take the view that their condition was self- inflicted and therefore they should not be given the opportunity to have a transplant ahead of someone who is sick and in need of a new organ. And it also may influence some peoples' decision about whether or not to put their names on the Organ Donor List. But, fortunately, or unfortunately (depending on how you look at it), It can happen occasionally that people with addiction are taken into hospital for a transplant in an emergency. It is quite understandable for any person who has waited for 18 months or so on the organ transplant list to be upset, annoyed and even angry when someone is taken into hospital for a transplant because of their lifestyle choices.

But everyone deserves a chance, don't they? Is it a lifestyle choice or is it an addiction that is out of control? Difficult as it is to get to grips with when you are the one who is being bypassed at these times, there are some people who unfortunately find themselves in a position of needing medical care because they have gone off the rails. These are the decisions doctors have to face on a daily basis. First and foremost, they are there to try to save lives. And personally, I think they do an amazing job.

13

Since Joanne was placed back on the transplant list, we were going to the hospital in Edinburgh every second week - sometimes more often – just to make sure that her condition had remained stable. We relied on my brother to take us through to Edinburgh when Joanne was too ill to travel by public transport. One Friday evening in July 2007, after a clinic appointment the previous day, we got the call to say they had a liver for her. The results of the blood tests taken at that appointment had pushed Joanne up to the top of the waiting list, and the call went out all over Europe to find her a new liver urgently. The transplant co-ordinator spoke with me, talking me through what they would be arranging to get us to the hospital and the timescales involved. She told me to make sure I had someone with me because they didn't know how things were going to go with the operation. I learned afterwards that she had been given only 5% chance of surviving. Good job she didn't tell me that on the phone!

We were picked up from our home by ambulance later that evening, by which time, once again, most of our family had gathered in the house, and were trying to keep us calm. When Joanne and I left in the ambulance the family members left to get themselves organised to follow us through to Edinburgh early next morning. At the hospital Joanne and I were put into a room where the nurses and doctors did all their final checks before the operation, which was scheduled for 8 am in the morning. I sat by her bedside all night, just chatting and trying to keep her spirits up. Early morning arrived and Joanne was prepared for surgery. I walked alongside the porters, holding her hand, as far as I was allowed into the operating theatre. I told the theatre nurse and anaesthetist to look after her, and left. As I turned away I was in floods of tears. I had managed to keep them at bay all the while I was with Joanne but now I couldn't stop. I don't remember how I managed to get back to the ward, but when I did I was an absolute mess. All my pent-up emotions burst free. After a short while just sitting there on my own, a nurse came in with a cup of tea, and to tell me that my family had arrived at the hospital and were in the family room at the front of the ward. I went out to meet them, and we all went downstairs to have breakfast. Needless to say, I wasn't able to eat anything, and that set the tone for the rest of the day. Although the doctors had said previously that some transplant operations could be carried out in about three hours nowadays, we didn't expect it to be the case for Joanne. So here we were trying to pass time til her operation was over.

I paid several visits to the Sanctuary in the hospital that day. The Sanctuary is a place of peace and calm, a place where I could pray and a place where I sought some kind of refuge from the reality of what was going on. It is a modern version of the hospital chapel, and in my experience was used mainly by Muslims for prayer. But it was a place where any amount of people of any or no religion could visit at the same time, and pray separately. There is also a book in the Sanctuary for people to leave messages about their loved ones – some good news messages and some not, but mostly messages of thanks to the staff in the hospital who were looking after their family member at their most vulnerable times. It is a place that I visited frequently during my many visits to the Royal Infirmary, a habit I had gotten into in every hospital where Joanne was a patient. Visiting places of solace at some of the most difficult times in my life. My brothers took it in turn to make frequent visits up to the ward to ask how the operation was going. Progress was slow, as we had expected, and it turned out that the operation took 12 hours just like her first transplant. We were sitting at the waiting area outside her ward when a doctor came along the corridor and asked if we were Joanne's family. That doctor turned out to be one of the surgeons who had performed part of her operation. His name was Professor K K Madhavan, an Indian surgeon who was performing his last operation in Edinburgh Royal Infirmary that day. He was leaving to take up work in Singapore. He is well known and respected in the world of transplantation, technologies and research. Everyone who spoke about him held him in the highest regard for the exceptional work he did, and he was sorely missed at the hospital when he left. Professor Madhavan had the difficult task of taking out the old liver - some believe that this is the most difficult part of the operation. How lucky were we that he was able to do this before he left to take up his new post. The second part of Joanne's operation was carried out by Mr Jim Powell. I never got to meet him that day, but he phoned my mobile phone just to update me on what had taken place and how things were.

It was later that night that I got to see Joanne after she had been transferred onto the Intensive Care unit. My brother waited with me, allowing the rest of the family to go home for a rest. My first sight of her was actually quite frightening. She looked so frail and so ill. I hadn't experienced that feeling previously after any of her other many operations. Usually my feelings were of relief that she had survived. But I was uneasy that night and I couldn't shake off the fear that I felt. Maybe I was just losing some of my positivity. I was getting older, after all and things were taking their toll. So I didn't wait by her side for too long, I was so overcome with it all, and so I left the nurse to get on with her job.

By the next morning, on my way into the Intensive Care unit, I was met by this casually dressed young man. It was Sunday morning, and most of the weekend staff dressed more casually than during the week. He asked if I was Joanne's mum, and then began talking about her operation in great detail, explaining that they hadn't closed her wound, and would need to have a think about how long they would leave her before taking her back into to theatre to deal with that. I thought it a bit odd, he looked like a young boy to me. Why was he talking to me about my daughter? How did he know all this? Then he said "Oh, I'm Jim Powell by the way. I did Joanne's op." I didn't have the nerve to tell him at the time what I had been thinking but you'll know what I mean if you are of my generation, we don't realise we are getting so old until we see the young professionals in highly skilled and important jobs and thinking they still look like weans!

I carried along the corridor past the security doors and into the area where Joanne's bed was. There was a young male nurse looking after her now by the name of Graham. He was an absolute star that day. It became fascinating to watch him, doing what he had to do, recording everything he had to record, ensuring Joanne was comfortable etc. AND changing his disposable gloves and washing his hands each time after every single task. He never stopped! And so kind and pleasant into the bargain. It was later that day that Joanne began to come to, and was gradually taken off life support. She was breathing only by the help of oxygen. I began to feel a little better, which was helped by the fact that when she really came to she wouldn't stop talking. I knew that she had had different reactions to different anaesthetics in the past, but this was the first time it had affected her in this way. There was no pain and she was in a happy place. She seemed almost euphoric. And she was talking like a budgie. It only lasted for that one day, but it helped to calm me down.

During her time in the Intensive Care, the medical team from the transplant ward would do a couple of visits each day. I can remember one consultant, Dr. Simpson, say to me "we have done all we can do, it's up to Joanne now".

Within a few days Joanne was transferred onto the high dependency ward and was making good progress. It was then that they decided they would take her back to theatre and stitch up her wound. It was another 4 hours of surgery, but afterwards she went back to the high dependency ward and eventually was transferred onto the Liver transplant ward in the hospital to recuperate further. Every day was a roller coaster. Bloods were taken every morning, and sure as anything there was something different wrong each day. But eventually, after tweaking her cocktail of medication several times, she was allowed home. Even after such major surgery, patients are discharged as soon as possible to recover at home, for fear of them catching infection in the hospital.

It was great to be back, but with the benefit of experience of her previous transplants, I knew within a few days that Joanne wasn't progressing well, and in fact she seemed to be getting rather unwell within these first few days of being at home. We had left the hospital on the Thursday, and I telephone our GP on the Monday to talk to him about this. He came rushing out to see her, but he said all her obs. were ok. But he hadn't seen her in the hospital so he couldn't comment on whether or not she was in fact getting sicker. We were due to go back for a check-up at the hospital clinic on Thursday again anyway, but he said if she got worse to give him a call.

She didn't get worse, but she didn't improve either, so I was relieved when Thursday came round and we made our way through to Edinburgh for her appointment. Joanne still wasn't mobile, so we were using a wheelchair for her to get around. My brother was driving us through for her appointments, so we managed to get there without too much trouble. But when we arrived, the nurse on the clinic, who had gotten to know Joanne very well over the last year or so, knew instinctively that she was not as well as she should have been after the transplant. She ushered us into a side room away from other patients and went to speak to the consultant who was taking the clinic that day, asking him to see Joanne next. When he came into the room, and without causing any alarm, he quickly arranged for Joanne to be taken upstairs onto the liver transplant ward.

There they carried out various blood tests and within hours it was realised that she had been prescribed too high a dose of one of her anti- rejection drugs. So she was once again admitted into the hospital to sort it out. She was distraught. Not because she was so ill, but she explained to the doctor that she had tickets for her and I to go to see Prince at the 02 in London that weekend! He just sat there open mouthed. "So sorry Joanne, but it will take a little longer than just a couple of days to fix this", he said.

Even while Joanne was waiting for her new liver, she was still arranging and booking things like places to visit and concerts to go to, although she was annoyed that she wasn't allowed to go abroad during this time. But this was actually a bid deal. This was something she had been so looking forward to. This was PRINCE! And to make matters worse, Saturday night's show was the last show of his stint at the 02, so there was nothing I could do to change things. Except by some miracle, the very next day it was announced that he was extending his stay and would be adding more shows there. So I was right on the phone to the 02, explaining what had happened and why Joanne couldn't come to the show she had booked for Saturday but asked if there were any tickets available for the shows that had been added. The girl on the other end of the phone must have been sent from God. Honestly, she couldn't have been more helpful. "What about the final night?", she asked. "Do you think Joanne will be well enough to travel by then?" It was just over a couple of weeks away, but of course I said yes. Not only did she give us VIP seats, one was free. I could hardly contain myself.

I was living in the hospital to be near Joanne. At that time, a small section was used as a "hotel" for family members like myself. As it is the only hospital in Scotland to carry out liver transplants in adults, there is always a need for family members coming from different parts of the country to find accommodation at this critical time after the operation. So it was ideal. I rented a room which had its own shower and it saved me having to look for accommodation in nearby hotels, which were very expensive for anyone who has to stay for any length of time. Unfortunately over the years they have had to transform it into a ward for the hospital to use as they were running out of space for patients. Anyway, when I went in to see Joanne that morning, she just burst into tears at my news. She wasn't long in getting better after that. So all I had to do was rearrange our accommodation and our travel, oh, and tell the doctors of course.

It was over a week later when Joanne was discharged, feeling much better now that she was on the right cocktail of drugs that suited her body. The doctors didn't seem too concerned when we said we were going to London for the weekend. We had to come back the following week anyway – weekly checks are normal for a while after a transplant. Joanne was suffering from malnutrition by this point and she left the hospital with a feeding tube attached to ensure she was getting the nourishment she needed. I had to organise this for overnight feeds in addition to what she was eating normally, so I was thinking that they probably thought we were kidding about going to London or that we would change our minds.

But no, on the Friday morning we got a lift to Glasgow Central Station. We were helped onto the train, along with the wheelchair and suitcase (which included feeding equipment and supplies as well as her meds and our clothes). When we got off at Euston Station, arrangements had been made from Glasgow to assist us at the station. It wasn't until I got outside the station that I struggled with the case and pushing Joanne in the wheelchair. But it wasn't long before two young policemen came to our rescue, and duly carried her down some steps in the wheelchair and hailed us a taxi.

After settling into our hotel near Hyde Park, we decided to walk the short distance along to Oxford Street for a bit of retail therapy. Me walking, that is. Joanne sitting back in the wheelchair and enjoying the ride. That shopping experience reminded me of the Little Britain characters Andy and Lou, with Joanne pointing me in the direction of whatever caught her eye, and yes, she did actually say "I want that one". She was enjoying doing normal things again and so was I. A new liver meant a new life. This was a new beginning for us both. It could only get better.

As it began to get dark, we headed for something to eat in a nice wee restaurant just off Oxford Street and then a taxi back to the hotel – totally exhausted.

The next day we chilled in Hyde Park, had something nice to eat, wandered round Portobello Road market and then got ourselves organised for the concert in the 02. At a taxi rank near to our hotel I asked what the cost would be to take us down to the 02. £50 he said. So I continued walking along to the nearby tube station! We were told by a porter that the lift would take us down to the platform, but unfortunately it only went half way and the rest of the way we would need to use the escalator. Not user-friendly for anyone using a wheelchair. Luckily there were plenty of commuters who recognised our plight, and were only too willing to help, one carrying Joanne down the escalators and another carrying the wheelchair. Honestly, no-one will tell me that people in London are too busy going about their business to think about anyone but themselves. We didn't need to ask. They just helped. The last part of the journey was fine, as it is on the new Jubilee line and it is wheelchair friendly. So we got to the 02 without it costing an arm and a leg and pretty much hassle-free.

Now, I'm not a massive Prince fan, but that show was something else. That venue is enormous, and it was great that we had front row seats. I am so glad Joanne got to see him just when she did. It did her the world of good, and helped so much with her recovery.

At the end of the show we had a friend, David, who came to pick us up and take us back to our hotel. David couldn't take us to the concert earlier because he was working – he worked in London as an ambulance driver at the time – but he was kind enough to offer to pick us up after the show, and gave us a lovely night tour of the city on the way back to our hotel.

The following day we made our way back home, with a bit of difficulty. I hadn't realised how much of a problem it would be with all the extra shopping we had bought. Despite that, Joanne was still looking at more things to buy at Euston Station! She was certainly making up for lost time.

At our next hospital appointment in Edinburgh a few days later, the consultant asked how she had been during the week since he had last seen her. Well, she said, I've had a few days away in London and went to see Prince at the 02. "Your're joking. You didn't actually go, did you?" he said looking from Joanne to me and back again – waiting for one of us to say it was a joke. When we confirmed it was true, he just sat there shaking his head. "Joanne, I know you are a determined young lady, but how on earth did you manage". We both sat looking at each other. "I had my mum" was all she said.

The thing about the whole trip was, it made Joanne see that she was able to do things that she hadn't done for a long long time. So she could see that she had a future, and she made up her mind that it was one she wasn't going to waste.

Once her weight was back to an acceptable level, she no longer needed the 4000 + calories a day she had been getting through the feeding tube, so it came out and she was back to enjoying her food. Gradually she became a bit more confident too, and was able to drive again and get out and about herself, so things were getting better. It was wonderful to see her getting herself ready to go out with her friends again, doing things she had really missed out on for a fair few years while she was so ill before her transplant. And she was actually feeling great, and ENJOYING life again.

14

I went back to work as soon as I felt Joanne was well enough to manage things on her own as she recuperated at home. After a while, we both wanted her to get back into the routine of living a normal life again. It was my role at this point to arrange things for a change, and we gradually got back to going on short holidays together and occasional spa or hotel stays. Eventually Joanne was well enough to go back to work too, and without hesitation she stepped right back in there, as if she had never been away. It was so good to see how far she had come, and how well she was doing The missing link for her was her dad, but she felt that there was nothing more she could do to help him. She had come to realise that he had to make the decision to get well himself.

Joanne was also back in her old routine of trawling the internet for places to go and things to do and see. Mostly her thing was music concerts, but she liked West End stage shows, and so it wasn't long before we got back to our regular visits to London for a show and a bit of retail therapy.

One of the first shows we went down to London to see was one in which her "hubby in my heid" was performing in was called 50 Ways to Leave your Lover. It was on at the Bush Theatre in London. We had never been there before so we had to work out our journey when we got to London. We had our map of Shepherds Bush, and it looked like the theatre was at the main square, so should be easy to find. We got the bus along and got off at the stop nearest the square. We walked along the street, but couldn't find the theatre. There was the pub and the Cinema, but the theatre should be here too – right in the middle. But it wasn't there – or so we thought! There was a door that looked like the entrance to a townhouse right where the theatre should be. We went into the pub next door and asked the barmaid where the theatre was. "Next door", she replied. "Yeah, that's what we thought, but can't see where the entrance is. There's only a door to a house there" Joanne said. "Yeah, that's it" she replied. We went back outside and tried the door knob. As we stepped inside, there was a small reception desk like you would find in a bed and breakfast establishment in Blackpool. A young girl was sitting behind the desk. "We're looking for the Bush Theatre" we said. "Yeah, that's us". So once we had established we were in the right place and told her we had tickets for the evening show, she escorted us upstairs in this tiny terraced "house". On the first floor there was a kitchen. Yes, it was a kitchen, but she pointed it out to us as the "bar". We followed her up to the next floor which she told us was the "theatre". It was the living room. Seriously. It was the living room of a townhouse in the middle of Shepherds Bush. It had two rows of (school) benches along three walls of the room, and in front of the remaining wall was the "stage".

We had our pick of the seats, and decided to sit in the first two seats nearest to the "stage" on the second (raised seating) row. The place quickly filled up, and when the play began, the four actors entered the stage from a side room. After the first part and to our utter disbelief Ralf Little sat on the front row bench right at our feet and did this every time he came off " stage" for the rest of the show. I have never seen Joanne so star struck. She couldn't speak. She was so in awe of him and being so close to her idol. It took all of my willpower not to burst out laughing. We went back six months later when they did a Christmas version of the same play! Apparently Ralf lives locally, and this was him supporting his local theatre group. The play did attract other actors along to see him, so we were sitting in the "living room" with the likes of Clair Danes. And I believe his support went a long way in helping the theatre group move on to a brand new theatre.

Over the years we saw many shows in London including The Lion King, Wicked, Jersey Boys, Mamma Mia, The Phantom of the Opera, The Ladykillers, Hairspray, and of course my very favourite, Priscilla Queen of the Desert. We both absolutely loved that show. From the minute the curtain went up the theatre was electric. The audience went mad for the show. It was just pure "showtime" and definitely has the feel good factor. We actually went to see it again several times over the years in Glasgow, Edinburgh, Aberdeen and Liverpool. Another show we went back to a few times was Jersey Boys which Joanne totally loved. We usually did something different every trip to London like visiting one of the Palaces, or a trip to Campden or Portobello

Road markets. Leicester Square and Piccadilly were always a must and so was shopping, whether at Primark on Oxford Street or Harrods (not that we bought much there, but it was always good for a visit). We usually stayed in a hotel in the centre of town so we had transport links to wherever took our fancy. London is certainly a place you can never tire of, but I am not sure that I want to ever return there without my girl.

Joanne was very much the motivator and organiser. If she saw something she fancied going to, she only had to say and we were there. She knew I couldn't say no to her and I was happy to go anywhere with her. She was my best friend as well as my daughter. She always made a point of treating me too, at birthdays and Christmas and not forgetting Mother's Day. Her treats became more extravagant, but she was working again and her gifts were usually trips that we would both enjoy. She booked tickets for us both to go see Paul McCartney at Hampden Park for one of my birthdays. I knew that she wasn't a fan of his, so she wouldn't be that keen to go along, but she told me she had booked an overnight stay at a hotel as well, a wee treat to herself on the night. It turned out that the concert was amazing and we both enjoyed it, as was the hotel, so we both had a great night.

She booked a week in Nice for my 60th birthday. It was an expensive hotel and I knew that the trip must have cost her a fortune. I had never mentioned to her that I wanted to go there, because quite simply I had never thought about it. But Joanne had done her research, as she did, and thought it was somewhere I would like. I couldn't help thinking that I wished she had discussed it first because I wasn't that sure I wanted to go there and that there might have been other places we could have considered together. So I wasn't really looking forward to it that much, but honestly, it was just perfect. It has everything you could want for a break away and all within walking distance. There is plenty to do and see in surrounding areas, and in the evenings there are loads of places to eat. The town is full of street entertainers, so the entertainment is free. It has such an amazing relaxing atmosphere, so once again her choice was spot on.

A couple of years after her transplant, we talked about Joanne getting her own flat again. She had her independence before, and we both felt it was important for her to get back to living her life as she wished, so we set out to look for a wee flat for her to set up her own home. She knew that she really wanted to do it but was a bit hesitant at first as she didn't quite have her confidence back but in her usual style she had to put her all into it and try it out. We had fun looking at a few places together but she just didn't see anything that she wanted until a flat came available in the estate just round the corner from the house where we lived. This was ideal. It was near enough to where we were living but I couldn't physically see it from the house and so she had her freedom and privacy, but knew that I was nearby. It was a ground floor flat with its own entrance, and she so enjoyed decorating and furnishing it. It wasn't long before she turned it into her own wee palace.

Things still weren't finalised with my divorce settlement, and I felt I hadn't been able to move on properly so that was the next thing to get sorted. It wasn't easy considering all the troubles we had been through and overcome together, but John had moved on so there was no guilt from my point of view. It was really difficult for Joanne, as it is for any child of parents who split up, no matter their age. She missed him so much, but felt that her dad had changed beyond recognition and there was no common ground any more. Although she had tried to meet with him many times in the past he would always cancel at the last minute. He was no longer the dad that she knew and loved. After a while, we got the divorce settled and so another chapter begins.

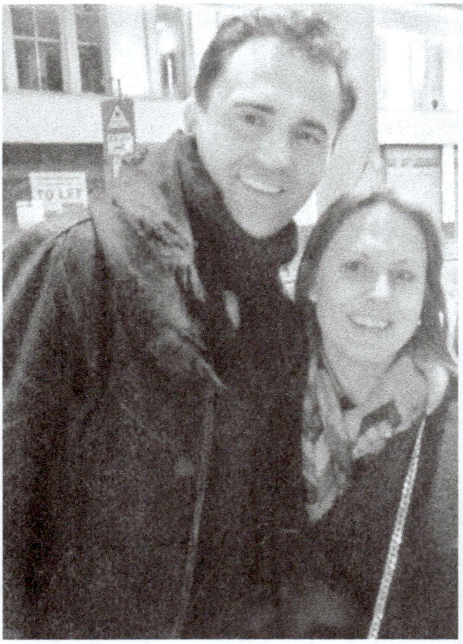

Met this guy outside Menier Chocolate Factory

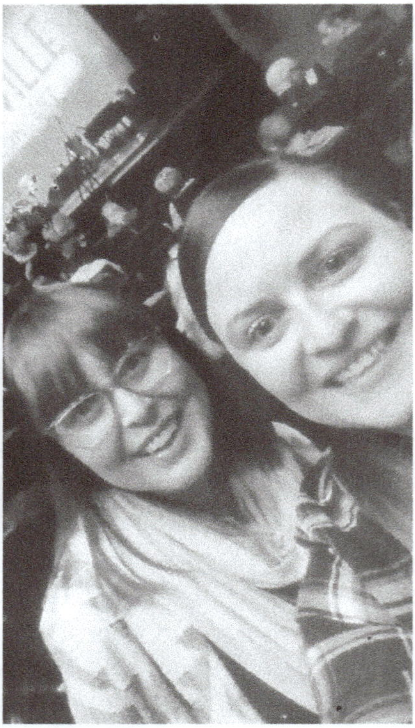

Karen and Me. What a night!

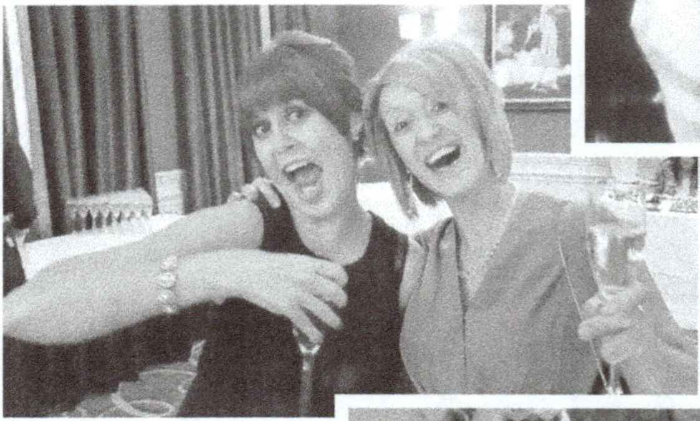

Heather and me - celebrating

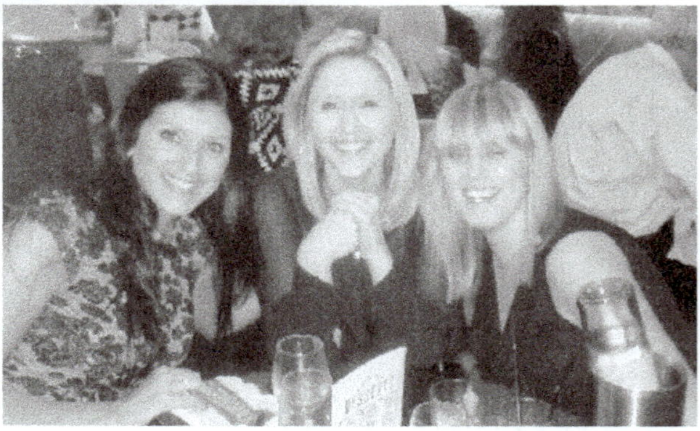

A wee night oot with Lynsey and Rhona

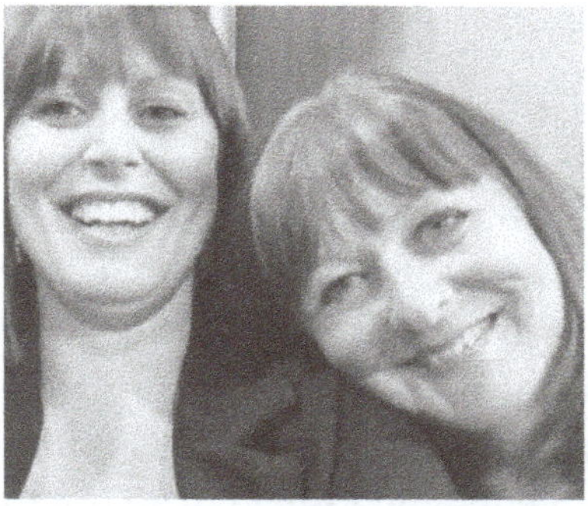

A night out with my Bestie - my mum

Me and mum at Gemma's wedding

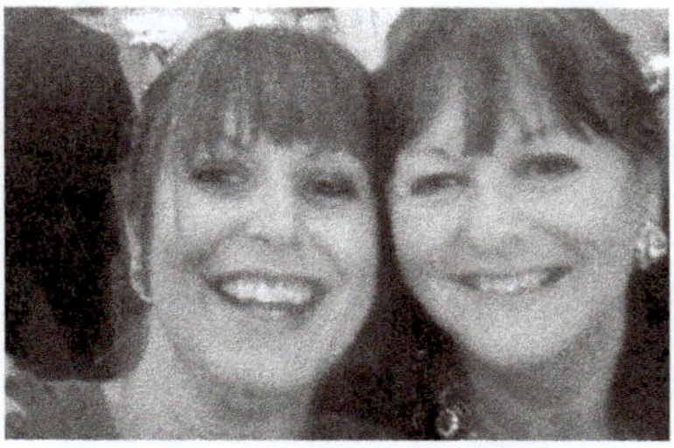

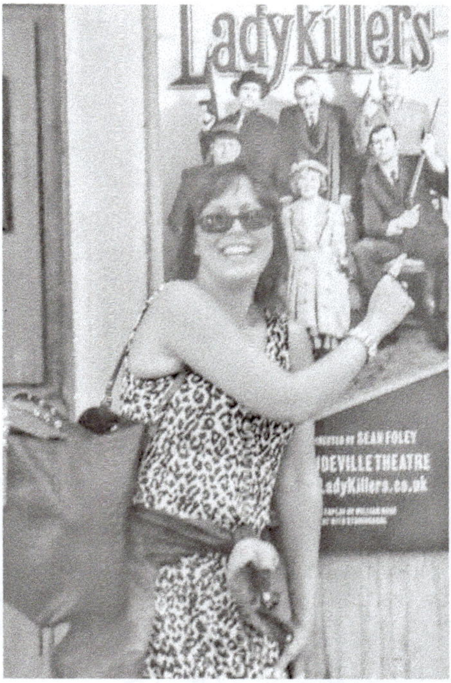
Ladykillers

Hubby in ma heid

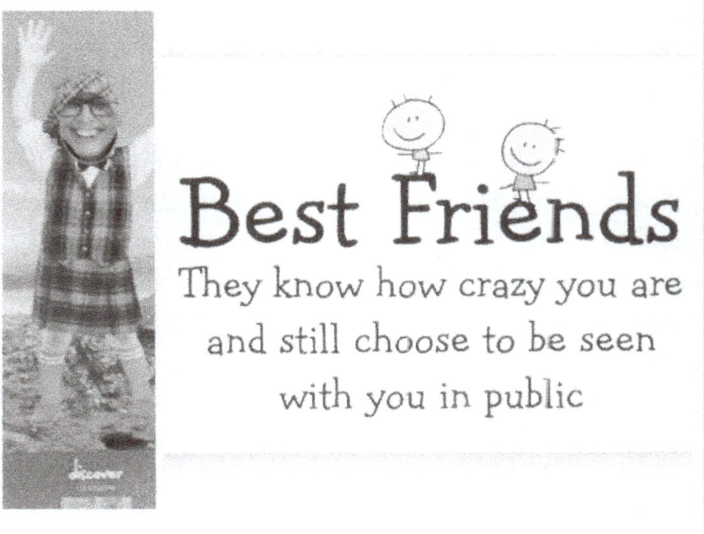
Best Friends
They know how crazy you are
and still choose to be seen
with you in public

15

It wasn't long after she was back in the swing of things that she began looking at holidays further afield with her friends. Her first long haul holiday was a three part break to America, visiting Los Angeles, Las Vegas and San Francisco. She went with one of her friends from work, Laura Bree and another friend Lesley Doyle. I loved listening to her stories about the places she had seen and the things she had done. It was a joy to see her looking well and enjoying life. I was so proud of Joanne. She was striking out for herself, taking control of her own world. She was living this new life she had been given to the full.

We still continued doing many things together. We went on two or three holidays a year, although for me it had to be short haul flights. So Spain, France, Greece and Italy were my limit! We went to London a couple of times each year too. We had many weekends away in other parts of the country. We took hotel breaks and most of my work's nights out, Joanne tagged along. She was my best friend and I didn't enjoy myself as much when she wasn't with me.

It may seem as though all Joanne wanted to do was enjoy life, which is perfectly normal after all, and more so for her given her medical history. She was so grateful to have had another transplant after being so seriously ill and weak before the surgery. She never forgot how lucky she was, and always said "the best chance in life is a second chance". She was now able to do the things she hadn't been able to do for such a long time. And she felt that she just wanted to do everything while it was possible for her to do so. She knew from experience that it could all go wrong again. So she valued life more, and wanted to make the most of every day. And she worked for her money, so why not?

Joanne also felt it was important to help others, and was involved with on line support groups. She gave regular donations to charities too, and just loved animals. Although I am not involved in any social media sites, apparently her facebook page was full of stories and messages about liver disease and transplants, and also about abandoned pets, mainly cats. If she had a quiet night in, she was often sat trawling through the internet looking at cats and dogs who needed rescuing and trying to persuade me to adopt one. Which we did on more than one occasion, but if she had her way we would have been running an animal sanctuary.

She also got quite interested in politics and loved getting involved in debates with friends. Tongue in cheek mostly. Because we all have different opinions, don't we, so there is no point in getting yourself in a twist about it. But we both agreed that thing we found most annoying about politics was the politicians! She was actually quite a clever soul, and wasn't long in sussing out that politics is a game to some politicians or perhaps just a way of making a name for themselves! Some politicians no longer seem to know their role. They tend to forget that they are elected democratically to represent what the voter has opted for, i.e. what they have said in their election manifesto. But once voted in, they seem to forget all of that. And they no longer have any regard for democracy. If we have a democratic vote on something - like it or not - voters have to accept the outcome of that vote. But for some obscure reason, some politicians don't seem to be able to do that. It should not be an option to have another election or referendum because you don't like the outcome. Quite frankly, that is just childish. Most voters haven't had their views represented for a long time now, but still believe in democracy. Maybe a different voting system would help? It doesn't make sense that one Party could have millions of voters voting for them but could end up with no MPs representing their voters in Parliament, and another Party could have just around a million voters voting for them and could end up with rather a lot of MPs in Parliament representing them. This is something Joanne and I chatted about quite a bit. We were never affiliated to any particular party, mainly because we couldn't agree with all that they represented. But we would often end up agreeing that the whole lot should be sacked because their behaviour in Parliament is disgraceful and childish – all they seem to do is slag each other off and nothing gets resolved.

It was a joy for me to have these conversations with her. I was in awe of her at times. It was something I never gave a thought to way back in the early years when we were living one day at a time.

But now it amazed me that she, as an adult, had the ability to work through things that she read about. Her logical thought processes were really intelligent and they certainly gave me something to think about at times. It's funny how some people are late starters, for whatever reason. In Joanne's case, I would never have dreamt in a million years that I would be having some of the thought provoking conversations we had. Not only about politics of course. As I said before, she was interested in the world, in animals and in medical care. I think if she had been healthy she would have spent some time in one of the third world countries, trying to help in some way or other. Or she may have been running an animal sanctuary. She often donated money to different charities. One of her favourites was Water Aid. It is inconceivable to think that there are so many people in the world who don't have what we in the western world take for granted – clean drinking water.

Another thing that Joanne took seriously was her work. She studied and passed her exams even though at times she wasn't feeling great. She loved the type of work that she did. She loved working with the "guys" that she helped as a Support Worker. She understood their needs, their hopes and their fears. But she also liked sharing the fun times, acting daft with them, playing their favourite music and singing along with it.

So things were on the up. She had her own home. She had a steady job. She was well enough to enjoy what she always wanted – a normal life! And she was so grateful.

But her miracle must have been the worst of times for the family of the donor. It was always in her heart and mind and made her more determined not to waste the gift she had been given. I have met so many transplant recipients through our many hospital visits, and it is the one thing they share. And yes, you could say the same for anyone who has had a life or death scare. But having been there myself, I do believe that for most organ recipients it is on another level – because they appreciate that often someone has died and that they have benefitted from that death. That thought can leave you feeling uncomfortable, and so the best way to show how much it means is to live your life to the full and to appreciate every minute of every day.

After Joanne passed, I received a message through my niece Leigh. It was from a girl she knew through work, and who had read about Joanne's passing in a newspaper. Here is an extract of what she wrote:

Hi Leigh, Sorry to hear about your cousin. I read her story in the paper this week, and again online tonight about how organ donation helped her to have the life she had. I have to say I had never thought about organ donation until the situation came about with my mum. Even when we agreed to donating mum's organs, we didn't realise what was involved. It prolonged our mum's death for nearly 24 agonising hours, but the organ donation team were great at keeping us up to date with what was happening at every stage, i.e, recipient matches, recipients being prepped for surgery, transplant team being there to transport her organs to anywhere in the UK within the timescales of the organs life outwith the body etc. We could have refused and my mum would have passed away within a half hour or so. My family who weren't already signed up for organ donation did so after my mum's death. I struggled with the time that we had at hospital comforting my mum until the medics said we could let her go, and kept thinking we should've just let her go when we were told she wasn't going to make it – what difference would that have made to us left behind, and she would have been at peace! We did receive letters that some of mums organs helped two women in their 60s have a new life after being on the register for over 2 years, but I think it was still a bit raw at the time and I neither felt happy nor sad about it But, getting to my point in this message that I have struggled to word properly and trying not to sound like a selfish git, is that after your cousin's story I am definitely going to sign up to organ donation register. I didn't know Joanne, but she definitely sounded like a fun loving, outgoing and loving girl that had the fulfilling fun life she had due to organ donation! Can you please pass on to your aunt that she made me stop and think about the way I was thinking about donation and thank her for telling her story and raising awareness about Joanne from the other side of the procedure. That made me change my way of thinking completely!

16

So Joanne was determined to pick up where she had left off. She couldn't sit still. Always planning and doing. Whether with friends she knew well or new friends she had made. She always had something to look forward to. Something to see – a show a film or a concert. Somewhere to visit – home or abroad, holidays were a joy. Dare I say it, were we becoming complacent? She often said she felt better than she had ever felt before. Everything was going so well. I can honestly say that I was so hopeful and the niggling feelings were being pushed further and further back into the back of my mind.

Still, the one main thing that was missing from her life was her dad. She had heard over the years through different friends and acquaintances that her dad was either doing well, or was really poorly. He had tried over the years to get his life back on track, but somehow he just didn't seem to manage to sustain it. I know that this bothered Joanne very much, but she knew from experience that she couldn't make him well, and that saddened her. There was nothing that she wanted more than to have him back in her life, to make it complete.

In 2013 John's family contacted to say that he was seriously ill in hospital. Joanne asked if I would go with her to visit him. He was in the Intensive Care Unit in the RAH in Paisley. When we arrived, we spoke with the doctor about his condition and we explained that there had been a relationship breakdown due to his addiction. When they heard what Joanne had been through, they completely understood why she had not been able to mend bridges with her dad, telling her that she really couldn't have done anything to change things.

For the next five days and nights, she was there by his side as often as she could be, taking leave from her work to do so. I would go over and meet her at the hospital after work. We were never sure if he knew that we were there. But not long before he took his final breath, he opened his eyes and smiled as we sat talking to him at his bedside.

It was a very distressing time for Joanne when he passed away, and all I could do was support her as much as I could and help her through this. Dealing with the death of an estranged parent is very complicated. It's not the same as losing someone you speak to every day. It is losing someone you SHOULD HAVE had that close relationship with, but had been robbed of it.

When a parent dies, it is devastating. You are changed forever. Yet in truth, Joanne had mourned the loss of her dad many years earlier and learned to make a life without him. But when he passed away, she still felt a million emotions in regard to his death. She was sad that she didn't talk to him on a regular basis in recent years. That he hadn't been in her life when she was fit and well. That they hadn't shared these good times together. That he wasn't there when she needed him at the hardest times of her life. She resented that she had lost the relationship she once had with her dad. It was different to any grief she had experienced when other loved ones had passed that she had been heartbroken by. That was uncomplicated grief. With her dad, it was messy. It was shocking and final. She was never going to get to speak to him, to see him as he once was – fit and well and happy. While he was alive, there was always hope that he would get well. That hope was now gone. Her grief was so complicated. She could go from anger, sadness, acceptance, shock, hurt, guilt, empty and resentful in a short space of time. It was exhausting.

She had always loved her dad. Of course she did. But she didn't like what he had become and she didn't deserve to be ignored by him during the years they were estranged. She resented his addiction and that she was always the one that had had to make the effort in trying to salvage their relationship, which she eventually gave up on doing. She was angry at herself for giving up, but she thought it might make him want to make the effort. But even though he did not reach out to her as she had hoped, she still loved him and accepted that his addiction was an illness.

Grief is a very personal thing. And Joanne had every right to grieve for her dad. While she was growing up, they were very close and had an amazing relationship. He was a very loving and thoughtful dad back then. Through time, her memories of him were more of the happiness they shared, and less of the bad times. In the early days of her life when she was growing up, his strength, his support and his humour got her through so much and no matter how bad it had become, she was grateful for having him as her dad growing up, for his love and support, for the life he had helped her live. She missed him every day he wasn't around.

Not long before her dad passed away, she was having some health problems too, and had been hospitalised for treatment of a really bad infection. Now she had to deal with the loss of her dad. She took it badly, and we spent hour after hour talking through things, remembering the good times and how our lives had changed so much. We had been a tight unit – the three of us. We knew that much was true. But we accepted that the amount of pressure we had to deal with over the years as a family was not normal, and we – Joanne and I - would just learn to live with the consequences of the hand we had been dealt. So we would carry on, and try to make some sense of this thing called life.

But with no real warning signs Joanne was catching infections and bugs more and more often. She would always make a good recovery, but by the end of 2015 she was looking really tired with dark circles round her eyes. We talked about it and as a result she asked to cut her hours at work to see if it would help. She had been worrying about her work performance, and it eased the stress of that a bit. But she still wasn't right. So, although all her blood tests were ok when they had been taken at her last hospital clinic in Edinburgh, we went along to the GP. She took a urine sample and this showed that Joanne had an infection. We were going to the hospital to the Liver Unit for a routine check -up within a day or so, so there was no point in taking blood samples as they would be done then. At the appointment Joanne updated the consultant, and he organised for several blood samples to be taken in addition to her usual ones.

The result of the samples showed that Joanne had Hepatitis E and e.coli. Most people in the UK will not have heard of hepatitis E. Until recently it was thought to be a disease only found in developing countries, but it is now accepted that the virus is also transmitted here, usually through food. Person to person transmission is uncommon and the infection is generally mild in its effect unless you have a pre-existing liver disease. The consultant said he would decide on a treatment plan, and would advise our GP what to prescribe.

A few weeks later, we were out at a show and Joanne complained of not feeling too well. She had just started on her medication to treat the hepatitis E, so we were unsure if that was the cause. We left in the middle of the show, and I asked if she needed to see a doctor or to go to the hospital. At the time she said she just wanted to go home and have an early night.

We went home to mine, and she had a cuppa and some toast, after which she said she felt a bit better but was going to go to her flat for bed. To this day, I don't know why, but I said I would go with her and spend the night there too. She didn't argue. That should have been a warning sign for me.

I slept on the couch, and went into her bedroom early the next morning. She was burning up, her breathing was shallow and it was difficult to waken her. I immediately phoned the hospital in Edinburgh. I wasn't sure if it had anything to do with the new medication she had been given. I was advised to phone for an ambulance which I duly did. The ambulance arrived with two ambulance technicians. As they recorded her blood pressure, they immediately called for a paramedic to attend. It took him almost an hour to get her blood pressure up to a level that would enable them to transport her to the hospital. When she arrived, she was taken into the resuscitation unit. I had travelled in the ambulance with her to the hospital, and was now sitting in a side room off the unit. After more than an hour, I was told that a consultant would come and speak to me about Joanne. Another hour later, he came into the room and closed the door. He told me that Joanne was gravely ill, and that the next 24 hours were crucial. She had sepsis.

Some time later I was allowed to go through to see her. She was hooked up to several drips, and it was clear that things were not good. I looked at her chart and read that she was admitted with blood pressure reading of 50/30. Apparently it had been much lower than this when her obs were taken in her flat. Although she had come through many serious situations before it still hit me like a ton of bricks. I knew she had a fight on her hands. But I also knew that if anyone could come through this, it would be Joanne.

I sat by her bedside most of the day. She was conscious and actually quite alert. The doctors were pumping her with steroids and antibiotics and other fluids to help her fight this infection. Gradually I could see that the numbers on her chart were improving and later in the night she was moved onto the High Dependency Ward. I was able to phone my brother to tell him what had happened and where we were, and he arrived at the hospital to sit with us once she had been moved onto the ward. So long as she kept improving, then I could relax a little and let the medications do their job and make her well. But it was a horrendous few days, waiting for my baby to come back to me.

It isn't easy watching our children suffer. The urge to protect them from anything bad is monumental for any mother. And so when they suffer, we suffer. And it hurts. And I think most mums and dads will agree it can be even more painful to watch our children suffer than it is to endure our own trials. Whether it's an accident, being bullied at school, a friend who hurts their feelings, a broken heart or a life altering illness, all of our children have to face the realities of life.

So what do we do when suffering strikes in our childrens' lives. Joanne had always had the heavy burden of poor health. But she was also granted the grace to carry it. I have never known anyone to carry such a burden with such courage. She had the strength of a thousand horses. My role as her parent was to support her to the very best of my ability. And my mantra was to never assign the heartache and despair I felt onto her. We depended on each other to get through these tough times, and somehow, we did.

So after a couple of weeks of heavy duty medication along with the love and care of the hospital staff looking after her, Joanne was well enough to come home. I still have her discharge letter. After listing all the problems they had overcome in the hospital, the doctor's final words were - I'm happy to say Joanne is well and is duly discharged.

Joanne came home with me to recuperate in her old bedroom at my house. We had both had a shock – her deterioration had happened so quickly – and we both just needed time to relax and recover at our own pace.

I had borrowed a wheelchair from the British Red Cross so that she wasn't going to be stuck in all day if she felt like going out. So we went out for drives and lunches once or twice over the next couple of weeks.

My morning routine was to check if she was awake after my shower and then go downstairs to prepare her breakfast and take it up to her on a tray. One morning I had opened the door, popped my head in as usual and I knew instantly there was something wrong. She was sitting up in bed, but she didn't look good. I asked her if she was ok. Her response knocked the stuffing right out of my body. "Just let me go, mum", she said - "dad's coming for me – just let me go".

I don't think I even answered her. I ran to the telephone and dialled 999. I asked for an ambulance, and although it was all based on my gut feeling and what Joanne had said, the operator got one to the house within minutes. It was a Godsend that we lived on the doorstep of the Ambulance Depot in Alexandria.

When they arrived, the ambulance team were not too sure what was going on. She didn't have a temperature, and her other obs. weren't too bad but given her medical history they decided to take her to hospital in Paisley. It was during the journey there that her blood pressure dropped dramatically, and so they radioed in to have the resus unit ready for her arrival.

She had sepsis again, so once again she was back on heavy duty medications and drips to save her life and make her well again. She was transferred onto the High Dependency Unit when she was stabilised and spent another couple of weeks there before being sent home again.

All Joanne wanted was to get back to living her life as she knew it. She had booked so many trips, concerts and holidays, and was worried that she wasn't going to be well enough to enjoy any of it. All of the set- backs that she had to bounce back from throughout her life had made her mentally strong and oh so determined to overcome everything that was thrown at her. But she had this feeling that one night out of the blue she shared with me – she wasn't going to get better from this! I was paralysed with fear and refused to listen to her. Although I had that sinking feeling that she might be right, I wasn't going to let her know. But she had never said anything like this before. Not once, despite all that she had faced. It was as if she had a premonition of what was to be her fate.

One of the concerts she had booked was to go see Carole King at Hyde Park in London. It was her treat to me for my birthday in July. We had it all booked, and at that time she was doing ok, apart from the medication she was taking for the Hepatitis E, which made her a bit drowsy a lot of the time. We talked about it – I tried to talk her out of the trip, but she was determined that she was going to do something that she would enjoy so we set off for London to see the show.

Overall, the trip went well, and although she wasn't working on full power, we knew that one of the side effects of her medication was drowsiness so it was no surprise that she was exhausted when we got home. We always believed that mental health plays a huge part on your recovery from any illness, and because of this Joanne was always in a rush to get on with her life, so she made a point of planning and doing things as quickly as she could after any illness.

But at this point, Joanne had had two hospital admissions at the hospital in Paisley due to sepsis, and was due to go to the transplant unit in Edinburgh for a check-up. We had already spoken about her upcoming holiday to America which she had been so looking forward to, and decided that she should put it off until she was much better. At the hospital visit, the consultant agreed that it would be best, and to be honest at that time Joanne's main goal was getting better, and it didn't seem to bother her that much about holiday. She had decided in her head that she would wait and go when she had fully recovered.

Joanne got her first negative result for Hep.E from the blood tests they took, so it looked as though all was going in the right direction. She was putting all her efforts into getting better. She hadn't worked since April, and had cancelled three holidays in total. She was taking care and not overdoing things and exercising her patience to the limit!

But by the middle of August Joanne was rushed back into hospital. Sepsis again. The doctors didn't seem to know what was going on. She had been doing well and started feeling much better, and then it all flared up again. The treatment was successful – full praise to the staff at Royal Alexandra Hospital in Paisley - but at this point we began to worry that she might have some lasting damage because of the recurring sepsis. The thing was though, each time she had it, it had been as a result of different infections. And each time she seemed to make a full recovery. So by the time she was having all her scans, she was on the road to recovery and nothing untoward showed up.

But it never let up. Joanne was admitted to hospital a total of eleven times over the months leading up to her passing. She had sepsis five times, and other problems beside. It was in November when she was admitted to our local hospital with an infection, and it was during that stay that she had her first heart scare. She had been having palpitations to the extent that it really scared her, but it wasn't given any serious thought as it disappeared after a while. On that occasion she wasn't transferred to the main hospital in Paisley, and it didn't develop into sepsis, so we both felt that her body was getting stronger and she was on the road back to better health. She was receiving medication for Hepatitis E – it had come back after her getting the all clear with three negative blood results. It was like two steps forward and three steps back, and the doctors were at a loss as to why this was happening because every time she was discharged from hospital her blood tests showed that she was infection free. It wasn't long before she was back in hospital again. This time she was back in the High Dependency unit in Paisley, and instead of being treated and being sent home, she was transferred to the Liver Transplant Unit in Edinburgh, to see if they could get to the bottom of it while she still appeared to be infected. The consultants knew there was something wrong, but they just didn't know what was causing all her problems. She was admitted into the high dependency ward of the Liver Unit. Probably the most expensive digs in Edinburgh, given the cost of all the equipment in her room and the staff looking after her! Again, after a battery of tests and scans, they could not find the source of her problems.

So, the night before Christmas Eve, she was sent home again – apparently well and free of infection. I had no food in the house for our Christmas dinner, as we thought Joanne was going to still be in hospital and the plan was for my brother Neil and my neice Leigh to come through to Edinburgh and spend Christmas day with Joanne and I in the hospital. So I frantically shopped and cooked on Christmas Eve in an attempt to make our Christmas meal enjoyable.

We spent the day quietly with the family. It was great to be home, and I suppose we were relieved that the doctors in Edinburgh couldn't find anything seriously wrong with Joanne. Fingers crossed, time would be all it took for her to get better.

The following week, we were welcoming in a New Year. We were both thinking the same thing – "Thank goodness that year is over – here's hoping this year will be a better one".

17

It wasn't to be. Not long into 2017, Joanne was admitted into the hospital in Edinburgh again.

By this point, I think we were both beginning to give up hope. Quite naturally so. I had lost count of the number of times throughout her life that we thought it was the end, and wanted it to be. The pain of watching her suffer was too much. But here she was, still battling. Don't ever say that Joanne was weak!

I had worried so much about her before, I was scared at times about her future, but I never believed that she didn't have one. I always thought she could get through everything and come out the other side. But it now looked like all the infections along with the cocktails of medications were having a serious effect on her heart and I kept asking myself "how is she going to get through this?"

She had to undergo a series of tests for this additional problem, and the outlook was not good. The cardiologist thought she would need a pacemaker, but she was too ill to have one inserted. Instead, they prescribed more medications that they hoped would do the trick. This was too much. How could anyone survive this amount of hospital admissions with serious health issues and still come out fighting. All my confidence had gone. I didn't know where to go from here. She was sick. We all knew that, but no one came up with a lasting cure for her persistent infections and it seemed like they were running out of options. To top it all, the heavy duty medications were now taking their toll on her body and giving her additional problems.

It looked like her premonition all those months ago was going to come true. My heart was breaking, but I couldn't let her see how frightened I was. I had to continue to put on a front, as I had been doing for so long by now.

By February she was sent home again with a clean bill of health. On paper anyway, everything looked ok and MRI scans were good. She was coping with the additional heart drugs, and she was put on antibiotics long term.

But, despite careful monitoring by the doctors in the hospital in Edinburgh and in Paisley, she was soon admitted back into hospital. She had sepsis five times during this last year or so. And to be honest, I could not understand how she managed to come out of it each time relatively unscathed.

Even at this stage, when she was discharged from the hospital in Edinburgh, arriving home at 9 o'clock at night – jumping into a bath while I ironed outfits for the next few days. Why? Because she was going to London the following morning! It had been arranged for her to go with her friend Karen to see Dreamgirls and another play that "hubby in my heid" was in on the West End. So Karen and her hubby picked Joanne up the next morning and off they went. I gave her extra money so that they would be able to get around by taxi while they were there, so that she wasn't tiring herself out too much. They had a ball!

She was also still making lots of plans – for when she was well again. She was booking loads of concerts with friends, and holidays for her and I to go to later in the year. She was spending so much time on-line, either booking things to do or posting things on facebook. Most of her posts were about transplants or liver disease. There were also loads about poor abandoned animals, mostly cats. And the politics – she was still sharing posts about politicians making a complete a.....of themselves. And believe me, there were plenty of those to be shared. But saying all this, I know that she was also saying her goodbyes to some of her friends. Probably at times when she was feeling particularly low, she would make contact with someone – her way of saying goodbye.

By her last admission into the hospital in Edinburgh in 2017, it was clear that she was dying. Her eyesight was failing, and she couldn't walk unaided. She was using a frame. Tests showed that she had three aneurysms on her brain which were causing the disturbed eyesight problems. Bad luck according to the doctors.

Her heart was failing fast too and I was told that there was probably nothing more they could do for Joanne. I didn't want her to hear this. I have no doubt that she knew anyway, but someone saying it out loud to her was not what I wanted. Although doctors think it is their duty to make each adult know exactly what their diagnosis and prognosis is,

I do not agree with it. I watched many many children recover quickly from serious illnesses from the time Joanne was born while spending time in hospital with her, and I believe that their recovery was helped by the fact that they didn't know they were sick. I believe that your mental state plays a big part of your recovery from any illness. So if she was to be told, I would tell her when the time was right.

But even at this late stage, after a meeting of all the relevant doctors and surgeons to discuss her case, rather than deliver the news that nothing more could be done, the doctors in Edinburgh told her that they were in contact with another hospital in Newcastle with a view to giving her a new heart as well as a new liver. She was also referred to another hospital in Edinburgh regarding the aneurysms.

So we came home – not to die, but to wait to hear if she would get another chance to live.

Within a week, a rather nice consultant phoned from the Western Infirmary in Edinburgh saying that he would like to see Joanne about the aneurysms and gave her an appointment for the following week. At that appointment they carried out several scans and eye tests, and made the decision that they could save her sight by giving her an operation. In most cases this operation is straightforward, but in Joanne's case, it could prove risky. When she said she wanted to go ahead with it rather than lose her sight completely, the doctor was full of admiration and said so. He told Joanne that he was in awe of her and that she was a very brave young woman. He was apparently a highly respected surgeon in his field and had seen many patients, so his words meant a lot.

We had nurses coming in to dress wounds Joanne had from being bedbound for so long, and to attend to any other needs she had. A new wheelchair was delivered so that she could get out and about. And she had the frame for getting around the flat.

She went to her last concert in Glasgow with Karen to see the Nashville tour around the middle of June. They were both big fans of the show. I dropped them off and picked them back up after the show finished, and they were both in high spirits.

A week later, Joanne had a massive heart attack.

She had a visit from the nurse that morning to look after her wound.

She came through from her bedroom after the nurse left, and sat having breakfast in front of the TV. just as another nurse arrived to check her warfarin levels. She had been on warfarin since her transplant in 2007, and had it checked regularly but because of all the changes in her medication over the last year, it was being checked every week at home any time she was out of hospital. She had gotten to know the anticoagulation nurses well over the years through going to the clinics. So when the nurse mentioned that she was looking so much better we felt that bit more relieved. It's hard to notice small changes when you are living with illness but for someone to say you are looking well and mean it, it does mean a lot.

We had been out the day before to look at a new sofa for Joanne's flat. She was anxious that her sofa wasn't comfortable enough for me to sleep on - well that was her excuse anyway. We had come home with the measurements of one that she liked and knew that it was going to fit where she wanted it to go, so when the nurse had left, she was straight back on her phone ordering the sofa. I had my back to her when I heard her say "oh mum". As I looked round at her sitting on the sofa, I knew instantly that she was dead. She was just staring straight ahead. And I knew.

I grabbed the phone and dialled 999. I was screaming hysterically. The operator was trying to give me instructions, but I wasn't thinking straight. I ran to Joanne and tried to pull her down onto the floor to give her CPR. She was a dead weight. I ran outside to call on her neighbour Allan for help and he immediately ran into the flat to help by giving CPR. I was still talking to the operator on the phone when the paramedic arrived. Apparently he was there within four minutes of my making the call. Allan took me outside to let the paramedic get on with what he had to do. Within minutes an ambulance arrived and I watched as the two assistants ran into the flat. A few minutes later another ambulance arrived and so another two assistants were there to try to save Joanne's life.

I was distraught. I was pacing up and down outside, talking to myself. I had lost my mind. By this time, other neighbours had gathered. One brought out a glass of water for me and a chair from his home for me to sit down. We waited – and waited. Time passed. It was over 30 minutes since the first paramedic arrived. Allan went into the flat to see how things were. He came and told me they were still working on her. More time passed. By this time someone had phoned my brother and he arrived. We were all gathered outside the flat waiting for news. I remember mumbling away to myself while people were round about me trying to comfort me. It seemed like an age before one of the ambulance assistants came out and walked to his ambulance. The other one came over to speak to me. It was then that I realised that I knew her as she had been twice before when I had to phone for help. She came over and hugged me, saying "the paramedic has done a great job". Joanne was unconscious and on oxygen when they wheeled her out in a trolley to be taken by ambulance to the RAH in Paisley. The paramedic came out of the flat and made his way over to his car. My brother went to speak to him and thank him for all that he had done. He said to wait for an hour or so and then phone over to the hospital for news.

I was so weak, I had to be helped the short distance into Joanne's flat. I began to clean up – just habit. Someone made tea. We were all in shock. It was so hard to process what had happened. I felt relief that she was not dead. I felt relief that she was being looked after in the best way possible. And I felt relief that I wasn't there at the hospital with her. I was also disgusted with myself. Why should my daughter be suffering on her own? I was appalled at my weakness. I had never let her go through anything like this before on her own. But I just wanted to fast forward and someone to tell me that it was all ok and she had come through this.

After a while, my brother phoned the hospital. He was told Joanne was in Intensive Care. Nothing more.

Later in the evening, we made our way over to the hospital and to the Intensive Care Unit. Joanne had been in this unit only once before during this last year and a lot of the staff remembered her. I spoke with the consultant, who was excellent at relaying all that had been done and why, and what the plan was over the next few days. Apparently Joanne had had another heart attack in the ambulance while being transported to the hospital, and was now on life support.

The next few days, I more or less lived in the hospital and along with my family we had taken over the family room. The staff were amazing, some telling me stories of the last time Joanne had been admitted onto the unit. She had sepsis at that time, but was completely lucid and many of the staff could recall the chats they had had with her many during the night when she wasn't able to sleep. They all spoke very highly of her. One in particular told me that she had ended up unloading all her troubles to Joanne, who had given her great advice and left her feeling much better. I was left wondering if there was any work getting done once Joanne got a hold of them!

After a few days, even the consultant Paul, who I hadn't met before, told me that when it was discussed at meetings with other consultants that Joanne was a new admission into Intensive Care, there were a few of them who remembered her with fondness from previous visits to the hospital. He had been a bit taken aback by this, telling me that it is very unusual for the doctors to remember patients in that unit – A & E, Intensive Care and Resus – as so many patients pass through all the time. But they remembered Joanne. "Wait til she starts talking – you'll know then why they remember her" I told him.

It was on the fourth or fifth day that they began to wean her off the life support machine. She was ready for it, they thought. And so she began to come round slowly but surely. She asked me what had happened, and all I could say was that she had had a "wee turn". I couldn't tell her the truth in case it would upset her. But she lifted the oxygen mask to say, "Mum, I am going to die". I looked at the nurse at the bottom of her bed. She said "No you're not Joanne, you're getting better". During that evening I was chatting to her and to the nurse. Sometimes, although she appeared to be asleep, Joanne would join in the conversation with a cheeky comment. She even asked if she could have a cup of tea! Thank God. She seemed as though she had got through this without any brain damage – something we all feared.

For a couple of days she was sleeping most of the time, and only waking up when she could hear a familiar voice. My brothers, Joe and Neil, along with her cousin Stuart were all with me most of the time in the hospital, only going home for short spells to clean and change clothes. Joanne's pal, Lynsey had asked if she could visit, and so she was with us too a lot of the time, taking time off work to be there. She was also brilliant at seeing that I had clean clothes to wear too! We had asked people not to visit, so apart from my friend Rita and Joanne's friend Hayley and her mum, there were no other visitors.

Hayley's sister Heather was one of Joanne's very best friends, but was on holiday in Mexico with her family and they didn't want her to hear anything about Joanne's condition through social media, so they had asked if they could come visit so that they were able to tell Heather first-hand how Joanne was. When they walked in the door, it was clear from the monitors that Joanne was excited to have them visit!

The doctors and nurses were hopeful. They said so. But the next day, as I walked towards Joanne's room I could see through the glass window that she was agitated. As I got to her room I spoke to the nurse who was looking after her. She said that her condition had changed and that she was waiting for the results of blood tests she had taken. I tried to comfort Joanne, but couldn't, so I asked the nurse to have one of the doctors come to see her. It was extremely upsetting for me – I knew that any change for the worse in Joanne's condition could not be good. I was panicking inside, but just then a team of doctors and nurses came into the room. The consultant took me outside to tell me that they would have to put her back onto life support, as her organs were failing.

I went back into the room, and held her one last time while she could still see me and know that I was there for her. It didn't take long for her to close her eyes, and I was led away from her room.

These wonderful people looking after Joanne had done everything they possibly could to save her life. They had been in contact with every hospital they could think of for help and advice on what they could do to make her better – hoping that somewhere there was someone who would offer to give her the organs she needed. But it was too late. She was far too sick.

It was the following day when the consultant delivered the news that nothing more could be done to save Joanne. It felt that we went from a treatment plan to this in an instant. I didn't question anything I was being told. I knew that my baby had been through enough. She was so tired. It would be cruel to make her suffer any more than she already had.

The doctors wanted to turn off her life support. I wasn't ready. I asked for a little time to come to terms with this. So I went back to her room and sat with her – just Joanne and me, alone together. I spoke to her for a while, telling her how much I loved her and asked her forgiveness for putting her through so much. All I ever wanted was for her to be well.

Eventually, I went to speak with the doctor, giving my permission to turn off the life support.

During the day, we had music playing in her room – Lynsey had made up a playlist of her favourites – Prince and George Michael among others.

Another bed was wheeled in to Joanne's room later that night as I had asked so that I could lie beside her holding her hand while she slept. By the next morning Joanne was still with us. The bed hadn't been particularly comfortable, so after I had washed and changed, I spoke with her nurse and told her that I wanted to lie beside Joanne in her bed. So the nurses sorted the bed out so that there was room for me to lie beside Joanne.

That night, Lynsey's husband brought his guitar into the private room after the consultant had agreed that he could sing a few songs. Kenny was a professional singer, and had been quite famous in his day – lead singer in a band called Logan. Staff had gathered outside the room while the family sat beside Joanne while Kenny sang and played guitar. The whole place was in tears. Staff

were hugging me and crying at the same time. No one had ever done anything like this before, and as the consultant said, it was our way -not the way of the hospital, and it was a very brave and beautiful thing to do.

After Kenny left, our Minister, Rev. Ian Miller arrived to say a prayer before Joanne passed. Then staff also left the family in privacy for the rest of the night. It was at one o'clock in the morning when Joanne took her last breath, me holding her in my arms, surrounded by my brothers Joe and Neil, my nephew Stuart and Lynsey, Joanne's friend. Joanne fought this battle to live right to the end. It upsets me so much still that her final battle was all in vain.

I still question if we could have or should have done things differently. There is still a lot of self blame and I carry a lot of guilt because of all she suffered.

Studies show that parents who lose their adult child are faced with particular trials, both in emotional and practical matters. It has a profound effect on your life. No one could have prepared me for this, the loneliest of roads. I had brought this beautiful being into the world. I had done all that I could to make her life happy despite her health issues. I did not expect to be in this position ever in my worst nightmares. After all, we were always buying time with every new treatment that came along that had helped her live a longer life. I truly believed that it would be only a matter of time before there would be a lasting cure. We had lived like this for the past 37 years. Grateful for the outstanding progress made in medical research before and since Joanne's birth. Grateful to the wonderful doctors and surgeons who had pioneered new procedures and miraculously patented drugs that would keep recipients alive after transplants. There was no end to their skills. And research is still ongoing. So why would I be any different to any other parent. Why should I not expect my child to live.

To have a child die before you, at any age, upsets what we all consider to be life's natural order of things. Children are supposed to outlive us. When it happens, your life, certainly as you knew it, is over. You lose your whole reason for living. You can, understandably, suffer depression as well as poorer physical health. It is a trauma that doesn't ever go away and you never stop wondering why it wasn't you who died instead of your child.

After a while, I walked out of that room for the very last time. I met the consultant in the corridor and he put his arms around me and cried. I was numb.

Joanne passed on 6th July 2017 – her friend Gary's birthday. Her funeral was held on 14th July 2017 – my birthday. I doubt either of us will ever celebrate our birthdays in the same way as we did before – Joanne will always be remembered on these days.

Joanne and I hadn't discussed what either of us would want at our funerals. She brought up the subject once when she was in the hospital in Edinburgh, and I shot it down. She said there were things that she wanted, and I refused to listen. I told her that we didn't need to discuss anything like that – she would get well again. And so she dropped the subject. I should have let her speak, and I should have listened. I didn't have a clue now what to do about her funeral, and I so wanted to make it what she would have wanted it to be.

The religious side of the service was as she had chosen for her dad. I tried to include things that were dear to her heart in the eulogy. The music was what I knew she liked. A recording of Rufus Wainwright's "Hallelujah" was played while leaving the church, and later at the crematorium Celine Dion's song "Fly" while the curtain closed on her casket. Leaving the crematorium it had to be a mix of Prince songs. Kenny also sang "Caledonia" at the crematorium, bringing everyone to tears. I'm told that I did her proud that day, a day I wish with all my heart I would never have had to go through.

I spoke earlier of the complicated grief that Joanne experienced after the death of her dad due to their estrangement, but I truly believe that losing a child is the worst experience any person can ever go through. You do not only have the distress of losing a loved one, but you also experience trauma following your child's death and because it is not the natural way of things. It is difficult for human beings to accept that this can happen. It's just not meant to happen that your child will die before you do. It is utterly traumatic – a truly horrifying event. The death of your child is followed by a more intense grief than the death of a spouse or a parent. This is the conclusion of many studies, and I believe it to be true. It certainly is in my case. I would go over the events of her last year on this earth every single day. I couldn't think of anything else other than what had happened. Watching Joanne struggle with illness and not able to do anything to make her well and whole again. Over and over in my head. All day. Every day. How all of my dreams and wishes had been shattered. How my prayers had not been enough. I cried a lot – every single day. It just happened without warning.

The parent-child bond is particularly strong in most families. It was for me and Joanne and early on after she passed, I experienced extreme levels of yearning and searching for her. From the moment I opened my eyes in the morning, the realisation that she was gone was there. I wasn't just alone – I felt lonely too. I found it difficult to get out of bed. Many nights I spent playing games on my tablet – my new best friend. Mindless games were all I could concentrate on. Quite often, I never went to bed at all. It was a lazy, pointless existence.

Grieving is exhausting. Your mind is full of the person you have lost. Nothing else matters – only your beloved child. Parents of children who die can suffer a broad range of difficult mental and physical symptoms, especially if they have a close relationship. In my case, I felt depression - accompanied with feelings of great sadness, despair, helplessness, abandonment and a strong wish to die. I kept asking myself "why am I here?"

Physically, I sometimes felt extreme panic and anxiety and also felt very alone after her death. I was numb and emotionally detached from life. There was no longer any purpose to my life, but yet at times I still found it difficult to believe or acknowledge what had happened. Some might believe that I must have expected it to happen at some point. But that could only be people who didn't know my Joanne. Believe me, no one expected it any more than they would if it was someone without her problems. She had proved the medics wrong time and time again. They accepted that she was a force of nature and were shocked by her passing. My life was empty and meaningless, and my view of the world was shattered. I no longer enjoyed life, or any of the things I once did together with Joanne. I say this as though I am "over it". I'm not. My grief is still with me. It's not better, but sometimes it is different. Sometimes I can cope a little better. But often, the despair and hopelessness overcomes me still. There is no such thing as closure when your child has died, and it is deeply offensive for anyone to suggest that there should be. I will live with Joanne's loss for the rest of my life. My loss is permanent. It is a hurt that can never be healed. Although the signs of my grief may not be so obvious, I will never return to the person I was before, the changes to my life are so profound.

But, like it or not, I am here and Joanne is not. So, instead of asking myself "why am I here", I had to ask myself "what can I do?" Doing nothing with my life was an insult to my daughter. After all, she fought so hard to have a life, and was determined not to waste a minute of it.

Even in my advanced years, I am physically fit enough to still get around and do things for myself. So I can keep my mind occupied by spending lots of time gardening. I can get out and about, visiting friends and enjoying lunch dates. But what can I do that is meaningful?

Well, Joanne should have been celebrating her 40th birthday this year. She had big plans to celebrate it too. But remembering how she got to achieve so many goals while she was alive, I thought it would be an opportunity to give something back. So in September, with the help of family and friends, I held a Charity night with the proceeds being split between The British Heart Foundation and The Scottish Liver Transplant Unit in Edinburgh. The night was also a celebration of Joanne's life, and it was encouraging to see so many of her friends turn up. There were lots of tears as well as laughter of course, and we raised £3500 on the night – while enjoying a fabulous night out. Couldn't help thinking that Joanne was there with us in the room.

REFLECTION

People that have been affected by Joanne's life and her death is a true testament to the impact she had on those she met and who became her friends during her short time on this earth and I have learned a lot about what Joanne meant to some since her passing. I am fortunate that they have shared some of their many memories with me, and it heartens me to know that she had such good friends who loved her.

From the early days living in Bonhill, Joanne bonded with the children next door – the McGuigans. There were three of them, John, Steven and Kelly. Fiona McIvor lived next door but one, and all the kids would play out the back garden or in each other's houses. From there we moved down to the town centre in Alexandria when Joanne was 2 years old.

Our new neighbours were Mary and Hughie McKellar, and they had a daughter called Mhairi. Mhairi was a day older than Joanne, and once they got to know each other, they were like sisters. The back gate that separated our houses was always open, and they both spent their time between each other's houses and playing in the back gardens. As they grew older, they ventured outside into the nearby park, and quickly made friends with other children living in the street, including Elaine, Lauren, Fiona and Laura. Mhairi remembers Joanne's quick wit and amazing sense of humour, and has admitted that she had almost wet herself laughing so hard on occasions when Joanne was on a roll. As they got older, along with their friends Elaine and Jacqueline (who was a great friend of Joanne's since they were babies) they spent lots of times together including holidays abroad.

Mhairi was with Joanne in our house when we got the call for her first transplant. She never thought much about Joanne being sick from time to time, but she has never forgotten that day. She remembers Joanne say to her dad that she didn't want to die. She remembers her mum Mary crying when we left in the taxi to go to the airport. She had never known up until that day that Joanne was so sick. Because, like most chronically ill children, Joanne didn't let her bad days get her down. She just got on with life.

In primary school Joanne was best friends with Gillian Grigor, but they went into different classes in high school and lost touch for a bit. But as true friends do, they could always pick up where they left off whenever they met at different times throughout their lives. Gillian has talked about many fun times they spent together including the hours spent watching films and listening to music that they both loved. As small children they were both close to their dads, and were very influenced by each of their dads' sense of humour. She remembers Joanne's knack of doing brilliant impersonations of characters from the telly or people they knew. She remembers her kindness and thoughtfulness to others – uncommon for children their age.

When we went to Addenbrookes Hospital in Cambridge for the first time, we were introduced to a family from Cornwall whose daughter had just had a liver transplant. Anna was a year older than Joanne, and had had her transplant a few months earlier. That meeting was to change both Joanne's and Anna's lives – they could relate to one another because of their shared experiences. They soon became friends, and were paired up to go on a holiday of a lifetime to Orlando the following year. Dreamflight has become an annual event organised by staff of British Airways who raise funds to take children on holiday who are terminally ill or have a chronic illness that affects their everyday life. Joanne and Anna were nominated by Addenbrookes hospital to go on the holiday while they recovered from their transplants. The girls got on great despite having totally different personalities, and over the next few years their friendship grew and they visited each other and spent family holidays together.

At high school Joanne made many new friends. There was Karen, Arleen, Collette who were all friends before going to high school and were now in Joanne's class in high school. But right away they noticed Joanne's bubbly personality and friendly disposition. They lived in a different part of the town, so Joanne didn't meet up with them after school. But years later they all became friends again – mainly due to Joanne's organising nights out. Karen remembers Joanne's determination to live her life to the full, and make the most of the hand she had been dealt. She never wanted pity. She was inspirational.

There was Heather, Hazel, Rhona and Lynsey. They met at high school, and became lifelong and close friends sharing many crazy happy memories of holidays, hen parties, weddings, birthdays and nights out over the course of 20 years or so.

It seemed that Joanne made new friends easily – she certainly didn't get that trait from me. I was actually a very shy person, and to be honest I only found my voice because I had to speak up for Joanne in the early days of her life. But Joanne could talk to anyone about anything. And she was a good listener too.

One group of friends she made included Nicola, David and Gary. Nicola remembers the first night she had a conversation with Joanne. They knew each other vaguely from school, and Nicola remembered Joanne as being a friendly soul who never passed her without saying hi. A few years on they were in a nightclub and Joanne stopped for a chat. Nicola was left feeling that she had been her friend all her life! She was so easy to talk to and so funny. Nicola introduced Joanne to some of the boys she had been hanging around with. Joanne got on well with most of them but Gary was as mad as Joanne, so their friendship lasted too. Later in life their banter on facebook was legendary.

Some of her work colleagues also became close friends. Laura, along with her friend Lesley, spent many holidays with Joanne as well as nights out at home. Janice and Joanne became close friends through work, and Joanne got to know Janice's family well too. Janice and her daughter Louise have shared many happy memories of their times together, although Louise complained that Joanne almost bankrupted her with all the concerts she would book for them to go to.

It seems that Joanne was a good friend to have. She made a night out fun, and always wanted her friends to have a good time. She was also a good listener and sensitive to people's feelings. She introduced her friends to each other, and never left anyone out. Even when she was sick and in hospital, she could make friends!

Children are very special to all parents. Joanne was very special to me and her dad – our greatest gift. She brought life and love into our hearts. I hope, as she looks down from Heaven that she FINALLY knows how much she was adored, admired and loved by those who knew her.

She fought like a warrior every step of the way to achieve all that she did and was truly inspirational. I will never forget her smile, the sparkle in her eyes, her witty humour, her loyalty and ability to love, and her love of life. She was a beautiful soul - inside and out and I am extremely grateful to have had her in my life for 37 years and honoured to have her as my daughter. I can honestly say that most of those years were happy times despite the obstacles we were faced with, and I learned so much from Joanne and through her. We only have one life, and I am not saying that you should live your life as she did. I just want to get the message across that anything is possible. Live your dreams. Make your own mistakes. Learn from them. But make the most of the life you have been given. I am and will remain so proud of my beautiful crazy daughter til my dying day.

Lightning Source UK Ltd.
Milton Keynes UK
UKHW021834150320
360373UK00004B/20

9 781908 898432